A CYBORG'S FATHER

Before you start to read this book, take this moment to think about making a donation to punctum books, an independent non-profit press,

@ https://punctumbooks.com/support/

If you're reading the e-book, you can click on the image below to go directly to our donations site. Any amount, no matter the size, is appreciated and will help us to keep our ship of fools afloat. Contributions from dedicated readers will also help us to keep our commons open and to cultivate new work that can't find a welcoming port elsewhere. Our adventure is not possible without your support.

Vive la Open Access.

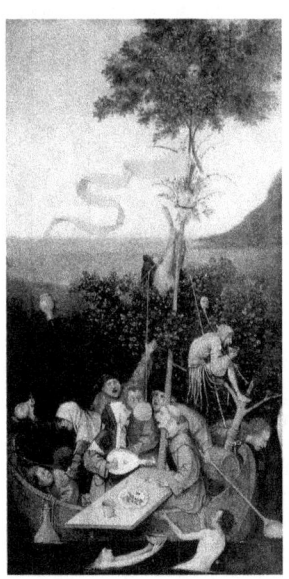

Fig. 1. Detail from Hieronymus Bosch, *Ship of Fools* (1490–1500)

A CYBORG'S FATHER: MISREADING DONNA HARAWAY. Copyright © 2025 by Dave Brennan. This work carries a Creative Commons BY-NC-SA 4.0 International license, which means that you are free to copy and redistribute the material in any medium or format, and you may also remix, transform, and build upon the material, as long as you clearly attribute the work to the author (but not in a way that suggests the author or punctum books endorses you and your work), you do not use this work for commercial gain in any form whatsoever, and that for any remixing and transformation, you distribute your rebuild under the same license. http://creativecommons.org/licenses/by-nc-sa/4.0/

Published in 2025 by punctum books, Earth, Milky Way.
https://punctumbooks.com

ISBN-13: 978-1-68571-230-3 (print)
ISBN-13: 978-1-68571-231-0 (ePDF)

DOI: 10.53288/0525.1.00

LCCN: 2025932606
Library of Congress Cataloging Data is available from the Library of Congress

Editing: Vincent W.J. van Gerven Oei and SAJ
Book design: Hatim Eujayl
Cover design: Vincent W.J. van Gerven Oei
Cover image: Dave Brennan

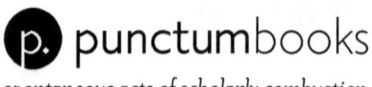

spontaneous acts of scholarly combustion

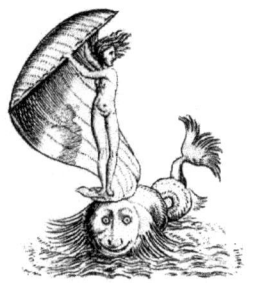

HIC SVNT MONSTRA

Dave
Brennan

A
Cyborg's
Father

Misreading
Donna
Haraway

Contents

Misreading · 15

I

Polemic · 21
Exemplum · 27
A Cyborg's Father · 31
Exemplum · 37
Turing Test: An Ambient Consciousness. · 41
Exemplum · 49
State of Emergency: Three Videos from Björk's *Homogenic* · 53

II

Polemic · 69
Exemplum · 73
Dancing the Machine: On Robyn's "Fembot" · 77
Exemplum · 87
A Cyborg's Father · 89
Exemplum · 97
Making Visibility: Naomi Wu · 101

III

Polemic · 139
Exemplum · 143
Singing Creation: On Mary Shelley's *Frankenstein* · 147
Exemplum · 157
Holly Herndon Creates a Life · 159
Exemplum · 167
A Cyborg's Father · 171

Bibliography · 177

Acknowledgments

I am grateful to the friends and writers who helped propel this book into being, especially Erica Cavanagh, Indigo Erikson, Susan Facknitz, Chad Gusler, and Michael Trocchia, whose early readings and encouragement were vital. I am thankful as well for the editors at punctum books, Vincent W.J. van Gerven Oei and Eileen A. Fradenburg Joy, for their editorial insights and vision. A special thanks to everyone who lent their voice to this book, near or far, directly or indirectly, to all those who live with chronic illness, and to everyone who works to make living with a chronic illness just a little easier. And to Kate, for every day.

The completion of this book was supported by grants from the Arts Council of the Valley. I am grateful to the Arts Council staff, for their time and kindness.

for A & K

Misreading

Syl. Sylvan, my forest song. My dark woods met mid-life. We cut you from the breathing trunk, greeted your bitch-kitty face. The first unknowing steps down this path. *"I looked up and saw no sky— / Only a dense cage of leaf, tree, and twig. I was lost."*[1]

At the end of your first year, we returned to the hospital. The machined forest. You were sick and getting sicker. You could barely lift your head; all day you lay on my shoulder, asleep or half-conscious. On our first visit to the doctor, it was decided the issue was viral and that all we could do was wait it out. Misread. We went again. When your pediatrician called in the late evening to tell us your lab work had revealed a blood-glucose level near 600 mg/dL, we set off into the night. Into the hospital, with its metal branches and snaking rubber vines. Its forking pathways, each a reflection of the next.

A rebirth. We fell again from the hole in the sky we all come from. We survived the hospital. We left the hospital. Swaddled in blankets against the cold March air it felt like the first time we

---

[1] Dante Alighieri, *Inferno*, trans. Mary Jo Bang (Minneapolis: Graywolf Press, 2012), 15.

walked into the world with you, only this time we carried both you and your invisible conjoined twin, type 1 diabetes. t1d.

Our world filled with sharp things. Syringes, lancets. And with bodily fluids: blood, insulin, urine dips to monitor ketones. Every three hours we pricked your fingertips to check blood sugar. Midnight. 3 a.m. To keep the twin happy, we jabbed a needle into the fatty flesh on the back of your arm seven, eight times a day. Filled repurposed laundry detergent bottles with used syringes, taped them shut so they wouldn't explode in the landfill. The pharmacy kept screwing up our prescriptions. Supplies scattered like our lives. One morning I woke to find a glucose test strip wedged between my toes.

The arrival of the machines felt inevitable. Because they existed. Because we were exhausted and tired of our fear, the constant second guessing, the not-knowing. Three months after diagnosis your first shipment of continuous glucose monitors (CGM) arrived. You didn't like the look of the thing, the orange and white device applicator like a cross between a vegetable peeler and Boba Fett's spaceship. You fought as we stuck the adhesive pad to your back; and when the applicator drove the thin filament beneath your skin with a sharp pop, you screamed. Then it was over. Within minutes you had forgotten about it. Two hours later your blood glucose readings appeared on a screen, updated every five minutes. It felt like a miracle.

Another six months passed before the insulin pump arrived. The addition of the pump to your body felt miraculous in its own way; no longer reliant on multiple needle jabs every day, we could finesse boluses previously impossible, non-invasively, administering insulin as often as necessary in amounts as small as the sharp end of a pin. All of it was small. Miniscule. The boluses. Your body. All of it untenably overwhelming. Looming large. We needed to be able to give you insulin in such tiny increments. How many times had we driven your blood sugar low with our clumsy human attempts at measurements only a microchip could feasibly manage?

And now you are a cyborg. You are four years old and have been living as a cyborg for three of those years. 75% of your life. The machines are imperfect, as the body is imperfect. We misread you constantly. Your body. Your devices. We read and misread the literature. Together we exist in a constant state of what John Keats called "negative capability," an aura of heightened uncertainty. Keats was referring to the reading of poetry, but the body too poses as a question. An uncertainty. The cyborg body a question best answered with another question best answered with a manifesto.

I like Wayne Koestenbaum's take on negative capability, which he likens to a state of panic: "Poetry leads to panic because you must ferret out the secret story behind the words. What if the buried meaning remains undetectable? What if the metaphor skein blocks your fingery entrance?"[2] How to savor this feeling of displeasure, is Koestenbaum's question, a question perfectly suited to t1d, to any chronic condition. How to trick the daily panic, the unsettledness of uncertainty, into a discomfort that doubles as a sensation to be savored?

The slow-boil panic of fatherhood. Of chronic illness. I will, I realize, likely make a mess of this father–daughter thing. Will likely make a mess of this cyborg thing. The mask of the technological. To paraphrase Anna Vitale, when seduced by the similitude of autobiography, we miss what we cannot see.[3]

---

[2] Wayne Koestenbaum, "On Panic: Whose Woods These Are I Think I Know," *Poetry Foundation,* July 3, 2023, https://www.poetryfoundation.org/poetrymagazine/articles/160534/on-panic-whose-woods-these-are-i-think-i-know.

[3] Anna Vitale, *Our Rimbaud Mask* (Brooklyn: Ugly Duckling Presse, 2018), 21.

This miss-reading, then, is an attempt at. An endeavor to. What? Learn what the questions are. Celebrate the mess. Take stock of the parts that comprise the cyborg death-life. To understand what I am or am not in relation to in my relationship with you.

This is to getting the fathers out of the way.

I

Polemic

While I write I track Syl's glucose levels on my phone.

This act makes me think of that masterclass advertisement, the one with the famous writer[1] who opines that the central obstacle to inhabiting one's imagination is other people.

Is technology other people.

When people & technology are simultaneous.

When my phone is charging the glucose app, Sugarmate, kicks the screen on every time a new reading is received. Every five minutes. Of course I look.

The body as numerical variant.

I regularly listen to the t1d podcast *Juicebox*. In conversations the host, Scott Benner, constantly plugs his sponsors, Dexcom (CGM) & Omnipod (insulin pump), citing their blend of functional & diagnostic capabilities. "The data received," he says. "The useful data." "The data necessary to improve your life."

---

[1] Joyce Carol Oates.

"The algorithm is the future of diabetes care."[2]

I attempt to think of my daughter as part algorithm. A data stream parsed by coded formula.

I can't stop looking at the numbers coming in.

I anticipate each update. Recheck my phone. Recheck my

daughter a graph of plotted data points constructed in real time.

I am often attentive to these data points in ways that I am not attentive to her. The diversion of care. While pushing her on the swing. While reading her stories. Ever removed from the immediate.

Blood glucose the unignorable other.

A recalibration of the invisible. An internal piece of her has, quite literally, been externalized. Worn upon the skin. Attached via pressure-sensitive adhesive.

Pump & sensor. Dex & Pod. We name them, like a slapstick comedy team

because I want to cry about it.

This cyborg we are raising.

The functioning form, the maintained form, status-quo form: cyborg.

The broken form, the radical form, the disobedient form: cyborg.

---

[2] Scott Benner, episode 252, *Juicebox Podcast*, August 12, 2019. https://www.juiceboxpodcast.com/episodes/jbp252.

In a photo essay on the hidden flaws we necessarily carry, one of my students described her own body as "broken." She was speaking of her tid.

A future artificial heartbreak.

The cyborg polarizes & propels. I attempt to come to grips: my daughter will always feel apart, like an assemblage of parts, yet also a part of: ever on the cusp of the human future, our transformation into biomachine.

I find hope here. Donna Haraway, in her essay "A Cyborg Manifesto," writes, "At the center of my ironic faith, my blasphemy, is the image of the cyborg."[3]

Is the image of songform. The blasphemy of pop, of hip-hop, the genre that is most purely cyborg, the turntable remade, manipulated to hold within its broken beats the improvisatory cadences of the human voice. We, ever more machine, see ourselves reflected in its form.

Songform. The musicians Fiona Apple, Robyn, Missy Elliot, and Janelle Monae (among many) all explore the experience of womanhood through the heteroglossia of the bot, the machine, the android, the cyborg. Within pop music's ready blend of digital & analog these artists disrupt the sexualized normativity of the leotard by adopting the discourse of the technological. They are, as Haraway notes, "made thoroughly ambiguous [by] the difference between natural and artificial, mind and body, self-developing and externally designed, and many other distinctions that used to apply to organisms and machines."[4]

---

[3] Donna J. Haraway, "A Cyborg Manifesto," in *Manifestly Haraway* (Minneapolis: University of Minnesota Press, 2016), 5.
[4] Ibid., 11.

"Our machines are disturbingly lively, and we ourselves are frighteningly inert."[5]

Jia Tolentino, discussing Haraway's vision of the cyborg as a forward path for feminism, writes that "women, formed in a way that makes us inextricable from social and technological machinery, could become fluid and radical and resistant. We could be like cyborgs — shaped in an image we didn't choose for ourselves, and disloyal and disobedient as a result."[6]

I think of my student, whose conceived brokenness has been shaped by the gazes of the ignorant, curious at the machinery attached to her skin, at the blood pricked from her finger, a fairy tale curse.

Who sees her body's radical redesign as impediment.

Who misinterprets visibility as affliction.

As father, I cling to the blasphemy of the inhuman as means of redemption.

As father, I pray my daughter machines from her body all its accessorized power.

From her illegitimate life constructs a singular origin.

May she be purely herself.

May she untether.

---

[5] Ibid, 11.
[6] Jia Tolentino, "Always Be Optimizing," *Trick Mirror* (New York: Random House, 2019), 92.

May she manifesto her hybridity into the insurgent truth, that cyborgs' "fathers, after all, are inessential."[7]

---

[7] Haraway, *Manifestly Haraway*, 10.

Exemplum

1.

In the ER. Syl's been screaming an hour. Three nurses pin her limbs. A fourth sticks her. Eight hands. Again, again. Dehydrated veins

collapsing. When they attempt to jab. A needle in her head. I step away. March the hallway. Labyrinth of laminated acronyms. -ist & -ism. Backward doorways.

Head failure. Veins too petite. Page the MRI. Magnetic like. Resonant like. Syl yells. Plenty of fight. Despite the DKA. IV in. We

begin. The bed is on wheels. I'm chasing the bed. Slow-motion footrace. Drop my face on the floor. Leave it face-down. Erased.

3 a.m. Brain's a drunk bird. Concussed, concussing. Words strungsung. Park the mattress in the PICU. Tiny body in a sea of sheet. Stormy calm.

Knees-to-chest asleep. While nurses swarm. Fix drips. Flick syringes. Tick boxes on checklists. Splint her arm so the wrist won't flex.

Somehow I'm holding. A Big Gulp. Suck the straw. Can't taste. & we are instructed: no liquid should pass the lips. Of the child dying to nurse.

A week spent. In pediatrics. They tell us get some sleep. We got this. But. The head can't nap. Pillowed beside your kid's illness. I'm a damn

giant. Sofa Lilliputian. Hallucinating. Nurses shirtless on horseback like Putin. Hospital slumber a petri dish. Bacterial bloom. Rotten chicken thigh. Clandestine tomb.

Syl twitches. Jump bedside. Door creaks. White sneaks. Formaldehyde whiff. Alcohol prep swipes. Test strips for finger pricks. Cotton balls to daub.

Cold air. I don my hoodie. Threadbare. Sunup. First day I wake up. With a new child. Inside my child. Twice

born. We live or we don't. Syl's tubes drip. Catch dawn's glint. Wisp of white hair. Mouth-breather. Lips chapped. Searching for their mother's breast.

2.

Bolus. Basal. Coverage. A1c. Tongues spit strange syllables, wonderland carousel of vocabulary. Barely slept. Head crushed. A sleeping

pill ground to powder. Snorted. Burnt nostril. Distorted olfactories. Drs. doing rounds, trailing residents. New nurse. New nurse. New nurse. Muted

saxophone emergency fantasy. Synaptic short. Post-op fluorescent hum. The huzz of horror flicks. Because I don't know. Anything. Because she's drowning.

EXEMPLUM

Poseidon infanticide. If I should kill my daughter. Via medical manslaughter. The culprits doubled: the cure the killer & the killer the cure. Twisted saviors, insulin & sugar.

A Cyborg's Father

We are in bed when the alarm sounds: a piercing electronic triplet, in descension. I groan awake. A dream? An ambulance passing? No, the noise is too immediate, too present. The alarm is not outside, nor in another room of the house. The alarm is in the bedroom, in the bed with us. It is coming from my daughter. My daughter is alarming. Is the alarm.

More specifically the alarm issues from her receiver, a cheap Samsung phone fitted with software specific to her CGM, the small gray oval adhered to her lower back. Beneath the oval a thread-thin metal filament nestles under the skin. Inside the oval a tiny transmitter signals out blood sugar readings. Syl is two-and-a-half years old. She has had t1d for more than half of her life.

Syl has shared a bed with us since her birth. We had just begun the transition away from co-sleeping when she was diagnosed with type 1. After that we gave up. It was easier to have her in the bed with us. To prick her small fingers, milk drops of blood from their tips. To administer insulin boluses. To slip her nips of juice while she slept. To make sure she was breathing normally. That she wasn't having a seizure. That she was still with us.

I fumble through pillows, searching for devices. Palm her receiver then her PDM, a second cheap Samsung phone loaded with software specific to her insulin pump. Squint into receiver screen: a sudden rapid drop in blood sugar. Squint into PDM screen: cut her basal insulin drip. If my daughter is part machine I am by extension a part of that machine. The cyborg's father is also cyborg. I am an operating system. I am a pancreas.

I tip from bed to fetch juice. Just in case. Syl prefers apple. Sleep-fogged I measure out ounces in old baby bottles, pour them into cups. I have become a system of responses. Once, in the days and weeks following her diagnosis, this moment would have been fueled by panic. Now I move in numb repetition, performing a patterned choreography void of conscious thought. A command in a script. Run program.

◊

Access denied. Can't differentiate. Collapses in a chair. Cuts himself shaving. The cyborg needs fluid. The cyborg needs a tune-up. The cyborg needs her blood checked. Dances up & down stairs, delivering. De-machines. Drives down the wrong road. Endless loop. Forgets the difference between. Forgets his wallet. Forgets his phone. Gargles vinegar. Human error. Inherent error. Kill process. Metadata drip. Misnames birds, plants, himself. Mistakes light switch for electrical outlet. Mismatches socks. Misses the toilet. Mumbles data into mantra. Overload. Proxy authentication required. Puts his shirt on backwards. Request timeout. Run script. Stares into the open refrigerator. Stares out from inside a refrigerator. Sucks the knife cut on his thumb. Undo command. Useless damage. Username/password. Vitamins in the palm of his hand. Vector attack. What's the difference. Why the body collapses. Why the machine redeems/enslaves. Yells silence. Zeros in on his corrupted file.

◊

I worry a lot. I worry all the time. My cyborg daughter tortures the cat in the living room while in the kitchen I am looking at my phone, staring at a graph of her blood glucose levels. It is the week before Christmas. A year ago exactly we were holed up in the hospital, Syl laid low with a quadruple infection (skin, ear, two respiratory). Now this week we have been struggling to understand why her ketone levels have remained elevated despite no obvious sign of infection or illness. Trauma flashbacks. All the time trying to stay out of the hospital.

While admitted, the nurses insisted we remove Syl's CGM. An inexplicable request we complied with. Because our daughter was sick. Because when your child is in the hospital you are desperate and the desperate follow orders, even if those orders go against what you know is best.

Stripped of her autonomy and hooked up to the health-care machine. Every three hours (or longer) a nurse came to check Syl's BG via finger-prick. When her CGM came off I felt as if a part of myself had been removed. Without the constant stream of blood glucose updates a sense of unease, of unmooring invaded. Knowledge is assurance. Data is assurance. In treating our daughter the hospital stripped us of connection, stripped away our intimacy, left us untethered, exposed. Imposed a process that displayed no concern for well-being.

If you have t1d the hospital is a terrible place to be.

◊

Are the machines working. Why are the machines not working. Is she simply very sound asleep. Has something gone wrong. His daughter, his cyborg: her origin found in the medical technologies necessary to maintain life: the machinery of needles giving way to wearable devices bluetoothed to touch screens. Herself a device. Input/output. He too is a part of the machine. A conscious AI. Monitoring, adjusting. He understands that machines do not require sleep. He attempts to insert himself seamlessly into the network. Awake at all hours, he worries about his fallibility as an operating system. About the precision of exhausted judgment. Is he the bug. He understands that machines do not worry. He attempts to delete worry from his files. Deletion fails: the pop-up prompt reads: Later/Choose. He chooses Later. He understands his role is temporary. His cyborg will eventually mature into a self-monitoring organism. Her machinery too will become increasingly self-aware. He longs to become an inessential part of the system. He worries he will be rendered inessential. At night, awake, the even breathing of his cyborg nearby, he observes the screen that controls her machinery. The shifting numbers on the display: he understands them as a form of normal love.

◊

Anymore I dream of structures. Empty architectures. In my dreams I am often outside, viewing the structure from a distance. The buildings tend to resemble those that fill the posts of the design accounts I follow on Instagram: cold, sharp, boxy, blank. Modern.

Occasionally I approach one of the structures. I climb the steps, open the door, cross the threshold. Inside I find Syl. She is always there, playing, happy. Inside this building not of her making. Inside this house where she must live. Because that is a part of the dream, too — the knowledge that this is a house she can never leave.

What I, this cyborg's father, want for her; what I fear I can never give her; what I fear has already been taken from her.

Yes, she must live in this house. She must. But as she inhabits it, grows into it, how might we make it more than just an occupied structure? How might we make it her strength, her armor, her insurrection?

How might we make it come alive?

Exemplum

3.

First time I. Stick Syl. With a needle. First time I stick. Syl with a needle. First time I stick my daughter. With a needle.

The vinyl on my mind's turntable. Skips. The circle's etched. Rhythm recast. Recording on time-lapse. Her tiny arm. My fingers.

Squeeze its fatty back. Nerve tremor. Immobile, Syl's weak, no protest. I tee needle to skin. *Flick your wrist,* says the nurse, *don't jab.* But I'm vexed.

Go too hard. Can't refresh. Syl yelps. Electric lurch. Mini syringe like a spinal tap. There's blood. Should it do that? Don't assume it

should. Nurse wipes the droplet. *You did good.* Insulin in. Syl's still breathing. Lungs locked in. Grooved. Peaceable. I collapse, cardiac. Need a shweet shot. Boozy schnapps.

4.

> *When's the last time you heard a funky diabetic?*
>
> — Phife Dawg

Big dorm freshman. Me & my friends. Hotboxed the room. Smoke thick, bass boomed. Every night listened. To the Tribe's *Low End*.

Hysterical. Movement. Tip had his fetish. Phife Dawg his butter, go. Back to the Busta, the old scenario. We sat in the abstract.

Open, fact-checked. *Theory* like a year of life. Lyric you can't quite get right. Now Phife Dawg's dead. March 22nd. Cause of death:

diabetic complications. 45-years-old, oh. *At least. It's just the diabetes.* Said a friend. When I told the diagnosis. KO.

Bell rings. Challenger with that O-ring. Just want to keep Syl safe. Not be left clutching keepsakes. Hold the terror near. Better fear than.

Same day we lost Malik. Same day Syl might have died. Sick wilt mistaken. For infection, viral. List the ways I'm thankful. Like Phife's voice. Endless.

Malik, please explain. This afterlife of rhyme. Tell me the future: does it keep getting smaller. A supercomputer looped. A stupid joke. Dead humor.

Are we a simulation. Disposable. Marginal. Are we the people who. Simply must go. You're alone, go. Ghost in your ear.

Can you hear it, go. Violent, brilliant. Can you hear it — O. A fresh download

5.

Fear comes at bedtime. *Sweet dreams* a deadtime. Sleep the endtime. Afraid to close. Eyes & transcend time. Popping Pepcid. Ache in the intestine.

Worry to the nth. Nights a red eye. All turbulent airtime. All attendant, no passenger. It's tech crime. This slow passing. Of time. It's this.

Count-to-ten time. Recite the end rhyme. Midnight. Time coagulates. The hour I etch. Time on the cinderblock of deep mind. Spend the most time.

Resenting time. What's the best time. To go against time. Erase time. By her bedside. Full minutes of still time. Eyelid dreams.

Straighten sheets. Hope she's alive when I wake. Remember in the morning to make. Apple muffins. During the bake-time. Grandparents to Facetime.

Turing Test:
An Ambient Consciousness

After Franny Choi

do you understand what I am saying

This is a Turing test. A Turing test comprised of questions plucked from a series of poems in Franny Choi's collection *Soft Science* that take the form of a Turing test. Questions that may or may not resemble the type of questions found in an actual Turing test. In the merging of forms (poetry vs. test) the very question the Turing test seeks to answer is amplified: can a machine pass for human? Can language alone manifest a sense of self into being? Can a program coded to respond to keyboarded prompts trick the poet at her own game? Or is the poet eager to be tricked? Or is the poet the machine, trying to convince herself, someone, anyone, that she is vital, alive?

We all want to be tricked into believing. That we are important. That we matter. That we are real. That our realities, that we, are more than machines asking themselves questions about the nature of their reality. Except that's exactly what humans are: machines who wonder. Who make possible all possibilities through bundles of imaginative circuitry. Machines who make.

where did you come from

From beside a cornfield in the wine region of New York state, in a small town on the southern tip of Owasco lake. The field stretched out behind our house on the edge of town, in summer a mask of green, in autumn a bumpy swell of mangled stalks and cobs. Beyond the corn sat a small grassy airstrip, a hangar with two or three single-engine Cessnas. Beyond the airstrip lay an abandoned train track, and beyond that a stream. On the far side of the stream a steep hillside jutted out of the lake valley. When the corn was cut, I followed my older brother back to the airstrip and watched him launch model rockets. After he set match to fuse they sputtered, jerked, then lifted high into the air, to the point of disappearance, before falling back to earth. When things went awry (misfire, explosion) we kicked through the corn remnants looking for the rocket's missing parts. On rare occasions we ventured back to the train tracks and picked our way along the wooden ties or balanced our way across the short trestle spanning the stream, water peering up at us through the empty spaces. Sometimes we dallied on the streambank, plunking rocks. I remember most sitting atop our backyard fence and staring out, across and beyond the cornfield, at the hillside I couldn't imagine climbing.

Also: Josh's tan stick-shift Volkswagen Rabbit, superhero underpants, Narnia, the field between, Charlie, Jell-o pudding mix, snow, Dana's basement, Tom's basement, the Pixies, Nintendo (the original), tomatoes, the Powers library, marijuana, Family Ties, cheesesticks, the county fair, Nikes, braces, Burger King hot chocolate and hash browns, Dry Creek, soft serve ice cream, Carrie, Little League, Rick's hand on my shoulder, Cape Cod, penny candy, Tina, Sonic Youth, the cherries out of Dad's Manhattans, mono, crawfish, saltines and butter, Biz Markie, etc.

how old are you

Today: 44.389. That makes me twelve years older than Franny Choi, who is a better poet than I will ever be. Who is younger than I will ever be. If it is young, it is good, the culture gods tell us. This fascination with youth, though: it should not apply to the poetic. Age and verse do not mix, the oil and water of cocktails. A poem comes when it comes. The vessel beside the point.

In the context of this writing Choi's age matters, however, as it places her in more pervasive and direct relation with the Great Machine during her formative years than was my own experience. The Great Machine being, of course, the internet, the inconceivable and nearly invisible expanse of metal and wire that instantly transforms anyone who encounters it into a cyborg. (I was in my late teens before the internet took up residence in my life. I didn't send an email until enrolled in college.) The internet is magic, and Choi, a queer Korean American poet, harnesses that magic to examine what it means to be alive as a woman in an age when machines are shaping not only our bodies but our minds. Choi writes: "Let me clarify: // when I say *cyborg*, / I mean what man made // the word for choking / on your own smell?"[1] The tension — between psychological and physical, of womanhood as social vs. literal construct, a being who is "manmade," the manufactured self crashed up against the visceral organicness of the flesh body — the stink of it. A disgust that arises from what humanity has made, or seems hellbent on achieving: a perfect, impossible form. The questions of *where* and *when* one is alive. What, exactly, is living? Who dictates the terms?

Haraway, as the collection's epigraph: "We are excruciatingly aware of what it means to have a historically constituted body."

As in: A cyborg is built more of the past than of the future. The future a blank page on which to tally the grievances of what has been.

---

[1] Franny Choi, *Soft Science* (Farmington: Alice James Books, 2019), 4.

why do you insist on lying

What does poetry have to offer a cyborg? Or the cyborg poetry? Most immediately it is a question of form. Poetry is a relentless form seeker. Beyond the traditional received forms, the sonnets, villanelles, sestinas, etc., contemporary poetry has made a game of finding formal poetic possibility in everything: grocery lists, parking tickets, online searches, flow charts, tweets, indexes, voicemails. Poems composed of first lines of other, unwritten, poems. Poems built of geometric shapes and hollows. Fields of ink splotches.

Soft Science straddles time in its typically untypical formal restlessness. "Chatroulette," a poem about the infamous website of the same name, is built of a crown of sonnets, a centuries-old form that finds itself bound together with android vocabularies, coding language, glossaries of terms, and poems made of phrases filtered through Google Translate, language butchered into slabs of text tenderized and strung with gristle.

In Choi's poetry the cyborg body is the past reconfigured. The cyborg body is a poem.

This may or may not be true.

do you believe you have consciousness

I am unsure how to respond. This question. I am no longer confident I understand what is meant by *consciousness*. An octopus (cephalopods slink their way through Choi's collection) has nine brains: a central brain in the head and one in each limb. How, then, does an octopus think? Are each of its tentacles separately conscious? What happens to its thought process when a shark corkscrews off a limb for food? And what do we make of the fact that an octopus can regrow lost tentacles? Is it regrowing a brain too? Is it regenerating an entire limbed sense of self? An entire consciousness?

A limbed sense of self: a branching I equate to parenthood. As a father I understand better the old cliché that having a child is like removing your heart from your body and watching it walk around. A heart doubled. Tripled. Quadrupled. The heart is believed to hold memory, and so might be thought to have a consciousness of its own. I am not saying that our children are like the limbs of an octopus, but I am also not saying that they are not. What constitutes a separate consciousness in one's genetic offspring? We do not think and perceive simultaneously, but we do not think and perceive entirely separately either. There are patterns, traits which persist in regrowth. Regeneration. Succession. Family a sort of octopus whose limbs float free.

Haraway asks, "Why should our bodies end at the skin?"[2] I often think of this in the middle of the night, awake and staring into the bright light of Syl's PDM, plugging in numbers, recharging her insulin cell. This connection between our bodies, genetic and technological. Where do I end, where does she begin? How far can the machinery of her body extend beyond her flesh-self? It is a strange truth that I could be on the far side of the earth and know her blood glucose level by looking at my phone. Wherever there is the internet. This oddly normal extended physicality: It is like her very blood has been put into circulation in the veins of a vast digital body.

have you ever questioned the nature of your reality

If this question means, have I ever desired to dissolve into pine needles layering the floor of the mountain ridge. To be sharp, flexible, soft. If I would rather be cloud or snake or thorn. If in the worn, redundant machine I find warmth. If, from the dictionary, I could choose only one word. It would be   It would be

---

2 Donna J. Haraway, "A Cyborg Manifesto," in *Manifestly Haraway* (Minneapolis: University of Minnesota Press, 2016), 61.

A CYBORG'S FATHER

and how does that make you feel

It is not that I desire escape. I have never been so happy as here. But the exhaustion. The small traumas of keeping each other alive. The soft sadness I am prone to when looking at Syl. Reading the posts of the Diabetes Online Community (DOC) has me worried for her future. The burnout. The apathy. The insulin rationing. The eating disorders. What other afflictions will she contend with? Isn't t1d enough? Watching her on the preschool playground she often looks adrift amongst the other children, like she doesn't quite comprehend how to play with them. While the other kids scuttle around her, shooting down the slide and back up, she stands on a high platform and shouts, "I'm growing like a pencil!" Sharp, to the point. Ground down.

how can we know that these are not simply simulated emotions

Choi: "you are covered / in smooth skin / a face it can trust / smile / even as you sense it / trying / not to blurt out / *monster*"[3]

at what age did you begin to suspect you were alive

I am thirty-three years old. It is my wife's birthday. A morning of teaching at the small college I am adjuncting at. End of summer, Virginia sun. The car is sauna hot, my back already breaking out in a sweat when my mother calls to tell me my father has died.

I don't know what to do with this day. I am as old as Jesus at his crucifixion. I am newly fatherless. I want to celebrate the occasion of my wife's birth. I am overwhelmed and numb. The car like a casket I will drive into the unknown. Born again as part mourning. A grief machine. In this moment I begin to suspect the day I become a father will mark the first death of an uncountable number of deaths that I have already died.

---

3 Choi, *Soft Science*, 69.

please state your name for the record

Proper names are fragile indicators of singularity.[4]

how do you know you are you and not someone else

Yes.

does this feel good

"What a cyborg wants is to work perfectly,"[5] writes Franny Choi, and as part of my daughter's cyborg system I too desire to work perfectly. In this task I have realized the truth of perfect failure.

The question, then, is who. Is failing.

---

[4] I stole this line from my book *Murder Ballads: Exhuming the Body Buried Beneath Wordsworth's Lyrical Ballads* (Earth: punctum books, 2016), 134, which I much later realized is tangentially about the presence of the cyborg in literature, the built body, the created form.

[5] Franny Choi, "What a Cyborg Wants," *Waxwing Magazine* 15 (2018), https://waxwingmag.org/items/issue15/21_Choi-What-a-Cyborg-Wants.php.

Exemplum

6.

In the voice of N, Syl's grandfather
Dx with t1d in November 1989, age 47

Hay made & in2 barn. Plenty of energy as school started again. Like God's calling on my life. Living in the country, growing crops, caring

for the earth. But especially teaching, being a dad. Didn't see it coming. Tired all the time. Pissing all the time. Bottle of oj stashed

behind the driver's seat in my pickup truck. 3 days in the hospital. On insulin right away. Hated to give up choco chip cookies but.

Straight back to work. Hauling lumber, hogs & cattle. Working on house additions. Running saws, hitting hammers. Didn't want them to know.

A CYBORG'S FATHER

Students or anybody. Snuck shots through my shirt behind my desk. Became a closet addict. A silence addict. Am I pretty upset about it sometimes?

You better believe it. But after 11,315 days. I guess 3 to 15 bad days is not so bad. So. What about faith? The God of the universe does not always answer

the way I would hope. As I prayed & believed. As I drove down the road trusting my truck to get me there. Thinking back

when I was a high school kid spring of the year. Plowing the soil with my dad's WD-45. Fire shooting from the exhaust pipe. Singing

at the top of my lungs, "Joyful, Joyful, We Adore Thee." The old version. Out of the hymnal. & it is the strangest thing after what's happened.

The things that keep happening. That even today. I keep singing.

7.

In the voice of V, Syl's grandmother
Has lived with N for 50+ years

He came home from the hospital. & got right back into his crazy schedule. He refused to talk about his diagnosis. Did his best to hide it.

Even though his younger sister was. Diagnosed with t1d at age 14. Their family never talked. About diabetes with each other.

N resisted any comments about what or when. He ate. I learned to watch in the background. Very aware that I. Who have been a faithful journal writer.

Logged zero entries during that time. I wrote down how many people we had for Thanksgiving dinner. Nothing about his diagnosis.

He always thought he could manage. Everything by himself. He never recognized me. As a caretaker. Or even a partner. In managing this disease.

It was stressful. For our entire family. His patterns of denial. He would push himself. So hard. When he went low. He often couldn't recall

what had happened. One day our daughter. Driving home from work. Saw her dad lying on the side of the road. He'd skipped lunch. Collapsed.

She somehow picked him. Up. Got him in the car. Got him home. At night I often sensed. N beside me. Sopping with sweat. Woke him so he could

get some juice. I always got up. To make sure that he followed through. When he was really low. He refused to drink anything. He would just shout.

I'm fine! I'm fine! At some point. I wrote him a letter. Of resignation. Regarding his disregard. For his own needs. I resigned. From being his caretaker.

Now I laugh at that. As if you can live. With a loved one & not do everything. You can to keep them. Sometimes he acts like he is tipsy.

When his blood sugar is down. It can be hard to take. Him seriously. Once, on vacation with the girls. A cabin in the woods. In the middle of the night we found. Him sitting on the bathroom floor. Chanting. *Boing, boing, boing.* It was so funny. Terrifying.

& hard for him. Growing up. In an extremely patriarchal home. To appreciate or affirm any kind of help. From us. To recognize any interference

or inadequacy. Which is how he understands his condition. I did what I could. The cookie jar. Was never filled again.

State of Emergency:
Three Videos from Björk's *Homogenic*

Beats on the right, strings on the left, a voice calling out from the middle. This was Björk's initial vision for her album *Homogenic:* a cyborgian merging of electronic and orchestral music, human consciousness at the center binding the elements together. The final album revealed a far more nuanced creation yet remained true to those first impulses. Sharp, skittering beats, digital flutters like pebbles cast onto pebbles underscore strings of "undulating fabric as flexible and durable as Kevlar," processed "until it's impossible to tell where the silicon ends and the catgut begins."[1] The triumph of contradictory forces finding perfect balance: repulse, attract.

Attract, repulse.

---

1 Philip Shelborne, "Björk's *Homogenic* Album Review," *Pitchfork,* February 5, 2017, https://pitchfork.com/reviews/albums/22835-homogenic.

Track 2, Jóga

> "state of
>
> emergency / it's where I want
>
> to be"

An island. Her island. Iceland.

The camera soars over landscapes otherworldly, ethereal, earthly. Rivulets like veins

feathered into capillaries, a frigid blood set in basalt flesh.

Rock moss ice.

Cliff sand waterfall

volcanic.

◊

Syl's existence a state of emergency. An alarm bell. Is it where I want to be? Yes: if it is to be with her. No: I hate this for her. Diabetes the island that reveals itself as CGI-replicant, unnatural nature. Is the grassy hillside that jerks open, the mantle's lava blood-boil glaring up, ready to vanish any life-speck that dares tumble in.

A heightened heuristic awareness. The body disobeys and so disobedience becomes a constant companion. The fault lines ever-present, on edge. Trigger happy. The body stutters along in blood sugar beats. Slips into cracks, unreadable. Makes of itself a flat landscape, a graph on a screen, bleating. The problem is one of surveillance. The problem is the body does not turn off. Correction: turns off only once.

◊

We stutter across geographies. In visual increments like a cursor's erratic tab across screenscapes. "Emotional landscapes," sings Björk as the rocks begin to bubble, the rifts stretch, the earth rising up out of itself in sliced segments, rendered divisible. What is indivisible. What cannot be taken apart taken apart in the cold complexity of the understanding algorithm. That is us. That is the chronic body.

"this state of

emergency / how beautiful

to be"

Is it beautiful? In the way the ocean collapses a cliff perhaps. In the way the wind uproots a tree perhaps. How the earth tears itself a new shape. It is beautiful it is dire it is circled around and born again and reshaped again and reanimated again. Iceland a young geography, yet unfurling its limbs. Syl so young and alive in the cracks and attachments of living. So alive in the hole of life misunderstanding itself.

◊

the difference between human beings and landscapes

is there is no difference

◊

Helicopter shots quicken. Rock upheaves, gasping. As we flicker between rushing ariels and claustrophobic underground shots, what is real blurs. What is photographic image and what is digital animation? What is the body and what is the land, when the land behaves like the body?

As the beats drop out at the song's coda, we find ourselves circling a mountain. A real mountain, an unreal mountain. We zoom in and a figure appears atop the rocky ridge: Björk, and not Björk; an obviously digital rendering of the singer, who is clutching at her chest, whose fingers have torn open a hole in her body. We aim for its center; entering we arrive at a revolving digital-green mass, like a heart like a tumor: an island.

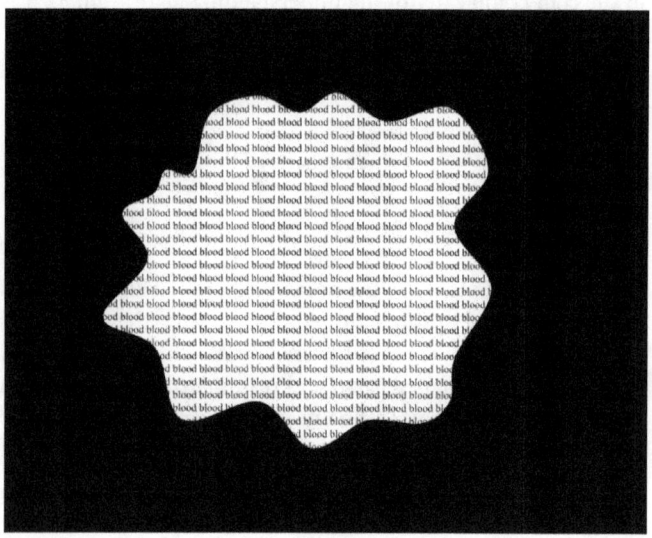

Track 1, "Hunter"

Syl, three years old, is a polar bear. In the bath she lays on her belly, limbs splashing, a swimming *nanook*. Because polar bears don't wear clothes she runs around the house naked, growling and crawling, scratching her parents' legs with terrible claws. Fierce, frenetic, and generally friendly, this polar bear prowls a landscape of furniture mountains and villages populated with elves, rabbits, hippos, dinosaurs. She is untamable, unknowable. When I ask the polar bear a question, she snarls at me, flashing fangs.

Syl, naked, gives me pause. Like any three-year-old she embraces the freedom, unembarrassed, a leaf in the breeze. For her the mechanical appendages adhered to her body don't warrant a thought. I can't help but see them, though. The insulin pump. The CGM. Lifelines. A visible reminder of both her vulnerability and resilience. The way they make a landscape of her body, crawling around her, every few days relocated to a new place, the shape of her changing, altered. At times they make me sad, but I don't hate them. I find myself thinking about how she will someday think about them. She jumps into my arms and my hand catches on one of her plastic parts, repulses, finds skin. These attachments. I don't know how to feel.

◊

The video for "Hunter" opens on a white screen, a snow field, as Björk's visage gradually fades into focus, her head doubling, tracers following her wagging skull before it crystalizes, sharp, uncompromising. We see her from the shoulders up. She is naked. She is bald. A newborn in an adult body. Something ancient echoes off her form, like a god adopting human shape. She occupies a liminal state, unmoored from humanity and intensely human. Human, and yet not fully a person, or so fully a person that she is difficult to look at, where are the filters, so when the silvery metallic scales begin appearing and disappearing on her face and along the dome of her cranium, it isn't altogether surprising.

Björk emotes aggressively. Her head and body waggle and wave, push from side to side, her face contorts unnaturally, the songform stretching expression beyond comfort. We are uncomfortable. Uncertain. As the video progresses the shapes and protuberances grow more frequent, more pronounced, Björk's face and body covered over with machinery that reveals itself in fullform as a polar bear, a techno-bear.

A human with an animal inside her. A human slipped inside an animal. An animal that is a machine. A human machined animalistic. Skin upon skin upon skin.

For three-and-a-half stark minutes Björk embodies Donna Haraway's cyborg-triad: the human–animal–machine fusion. The video is *haiku:* three elements, attempting to ask the question in the most interesting way possible. Paul White, director of the video, said of its concept, "the beauty of 'Hunter' is its utter simplicity. It's about a woman who allows the animal within to take over when necessary."[2] The publication *Freeze Frame* wrote: "It's about shedding the denial and embracing what we are — what we really are, even though it's sometimes hard to tell."[3]

It is sometimes hard to tell.

◊

Björk said of her polar bear, "they're very cuddly and cute and quite calm, but if they meet you they can be very strong."[4] I think of this as Syl prowls the house in shorn-bear mode, fingers bent into razor rakes, a head full of bright curls, smile cracking her undomesticated, polar demeanor. Think of this every time we jab something sharp into her skin, spotting blood, and she bears it with tight lips and a shiver. "That wasn't so bad," she will say. How we hurt her to protect her.

Or she howls.

Or she hides inside her fabulation, pure and wrapped in the skin of the hunting predator, a swift swipe of the claw away from spilled blood.

---

2 "Hunter," *Björk & Family Tree,* http://bjorknet.altervista.org/restored/10/.
3 Ibid.
4 "The Always Uncjorked Björk!," interview with John Savage, *Interview Magazine* (1995), http://bjork.fr/Interview-1995,982.

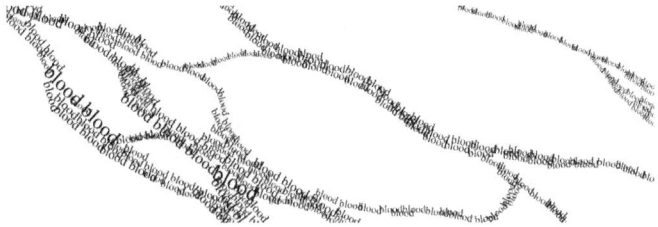

Track 10, "All Is Full of Love"

I first heard *Homogenic* in college. Sitting on the floor of my room, eating a molasses cookie, my housemate Chris walked in and tossed a CD in my lap. I put my cookie on it. Chris stared at the jewel-case plate for a moment then sat down in front of me. Through the lenses of his glasses his pupils like black holes, LSD-dilated. "You have to listen to this," he said, tapping the plastic. "I think you'll like it. I really, really think you'll like it." Acid enthusiasm. Chris's room was across the hall from mine; through our open doors I could see a canvas propped against the wall, the painting in progress of an old steam locomotive taking flight, the arrow of its cattle-catcher aimed straight at the bull's-eye of a full moon. His room full of paintings dominated by a series of oil renderings of hands, joints and palms and knuckles in vibrant close-up, captured in an almost violently inhuman palette of colors. Traffic-cone orange. Young basil green. Rhinoceros purple. Chris picked up my cookie and finished it off in a single bite, then scuttered away to continue his trip in solitude.

I did really like that CD. A lot. Björk on the cover in her sci-fi kimono, all frigid silvers and bloody reds. I liked it all except for the last track, "All Is Full of Love." Its beatless drift and muted monastic spaces felt too sugary, too blissed-out, too resolute, too swan-like on the heels of the tectonic angst of "Pluto." It felt unremarkable, like elements were missing. Or maybe I just missed the beats. I listened to that disc hard for several weeks, till Chris wanted it back. Then I forgot about it.

A CYBORG'S FATHER

A year later, maybe more, in a friend's car, "All Is Full of Love" reemerged. His one hand light on the steering wheel, the other cracked open the plastic case and slid the CD into the stereo. I recognized the opening track immediately, only it wasn't the track I knew. It had beats. Rhythm. The instrumentation was different. I loved it. This was the version I wanted to close out the album. I scanned the track list.

1. All Is Full of Love (Video Version)
2. All Is Full of Love (Funkstörung Exclusive Mix)
3. All Is Full of Love (Strings)
4. All Is Full of Love (Album Version)
5. All Is Full of Love (Plaid Mix)
6. All Is Full of Love (Guy Sigsworth Mix)[5]

As the Video Version segued into the Funkstörung Exclusive Mix, the song emerged as something other entirely, the track's stems chopped and pasted into a companion species that felt unrecognizable from its origin yet maintained a genetic spiritual throughline. The song in this guise sounded coldly modern and family familiar, as if the sleek corridors of a business conglomerate's financial headquarters had mated with the creaky orifices of your grandparents' old farmhouse. "I thought I hated this song," I said. "Have you seen the video?" my friend said. "It'll blow your mind."

The video is a masterwork of frigid sensuality. It consists, in brief, of two robots, both wearing molded porcelain versions of Björk's face, making out while robotic factory arms hover around them and squirt milky-white lube liquid into their working parts. Chris Cunningham, the director, said when he first heard the track he wrote down the words "sexual," "white porcelain," "milk," and "surgery." Björk brought to their first meeting a book of Chinese Kama Sutra prints as a visual refer-

---

5   Björk, *All Is Full of Love* (US CD single) (Elektra Records, 1999).

ence. "I got to play around with the two things I was into as a teenager," Cunningham said, "robots and porn."[6]

The sexual focus of the visual surprised me. I had always heard the song more as an ode to spiritual transcendence; the Buddhist principles of kindness, compassion, joy, and equanimity seemed to radiate out of its synth-string smoothness. All is full of love. Yes. Perhaps this feeling is why Björk chose the Howie B. remix of the track for the album; its fragile sense of wholeness and newness make the perfect end for an opus full of the tortured nerve endings inherent in fitting together parts that don't naturally meld, whether sonically or relationally. The cyborg is not born without pain.

Nor is the album version of the song Björk's original. The original is the video version, the one Cunningham heard, the one that accompanies the Björk-bots in their stoic kiss. The one that got me all excited in the car. The one whose molasses beats and glistening glissandos are woozy with the transcendence of bodily pleasure. All is full of love, yes, in that we are robots programmed to mate and mate and mate: to reproduce. We comprise the industrial production line of ourselves.[7]

◊

Cunningham's original treatment for the video, in full:

> Against black we hear the faint sound of electricity gently surging. All around us, banks of fluorescent lights, behind Plexiglas flicker to life at random, illuminating an elegant,

---

[6] "All Is Full of Love," *Björk Wiki*, https://björk.fandom.com/wiki/All_Is_Full_of_Love_(song).

[7] It is worth emphasizing that the two bots in the video are both Björk. In that way the video scans as frighteningly prescient, in this age of self-help and self-love. In contrast to Haraway's emphasis on interdependence, here is the ultimate danger of staring too long at ourselves — self-love becomes the only type of love that stirs us.

pristine white environment. It has a Japanese feel to it, a simplicity in its design. As we track forwards we are dwarfed on either side by two enormous medical/industrial robots. In unison they sweep around towards a workspace littered with eggshell-white plastic parts. As we get closer the parts become more visible and reveal an organic nature, their shapes resemble humanoid forms. From above we see clearly a female form in a fetal position completely abstracted and disassembled. Although it is artificial it is beautiful and elegant. The machines set to work in extreme slow motion. Their arms gracefully engaging with the incomplete human form, removing and adding parts to the partially hollow plastic shell and its matte black complex inner workings. Although only the front portion is in place its features are clearly those of Björk's, albeit the smoothed panels of a Japanese motorbike. The eyes open as the robotic arms construct consciousness. Warm orange sparks fly against the cold blue white plastic. It feels like we are watching the last stages of an artificial intelligence's birth. As it starts to sing, the elegance of the song and the imagery is contrasted by the abstractions caused by this incomplete form. It never quite becomes whole. As the track unfolds so too does the imagery developing in stages. The figure, still incomplete, is upright now. Its hand reaching up to touch its own face. We reveal more of the scene. Gently white fluid, like milk, starts to wash over the form and eventually engulfs it (this would be achieved by submerging the forms in a vat of milk and draining it off, filmed in reverse). When the form emerges from the vat we reveal that it is number two in a series. Still with Björk's features, the two ARTIFICIAL INTELLIGENCES begin to engage with one another. Locked together in a surreal embrace, parts intertwined and fused, we concentrate now on details, kissing, slow motion white fluid, fluorescent light. The imagery is slowly becoming more sexual but way too surreal and abstract to be offensive. We see the plastic bodies begin to unfold like strange flowers. The last sequence of shots as we pull back very wide reveal an indescribably abstract life form made from the two unfolded, artificial, humanoid forms. It's like Kama Sutra meets Industrial Robotics. The shots in this video will not be as difficult as you might imagine. The main performance aspect of the video would involve attaching blue panels to Björk's body and replacing these areas with model parts filmed against the same background. This will give the illusion of her being hollow, completely artificial. We would shoot everything as a lock off. As we approach the finale, the shots would possibly start to include a mixture of computer graphics and live action, used seamlessly to depict these robots unfolding. A lot of preparatory work would be needed and some compositing, but the shot would be very simple. I am convinced that this would make an extraordinary surreal performance video. The imagery would be majestic, and we could be as sexually suggestive as we like and get away with it.[8]

Björk channels Haraway's notion that bodies are created rather than born.[9] Of earth, animal, machine, a woman builds and is built. The artist builds and is built. Humans build and are built: we alter landscapes, adopt other species as our children, reform our physicality with tech designed to optimize and support life. Björk is built of the stories she tells through song and film; a composite creature, a self un(st)able to realize its selfhood without utilizing the attachments available that make life livable; a piece of built technology that sheds its human skin and is reborn in a skin unmistakably (un)human.

◊

---

8 "All Is Full of Love," *Björk Wiki*.
9 Donna J. Haraway, "A Cyborg Manifesto," in *Manifestly Haraway* (Minneapolis: University of Minnesota Press, 2016), 65.

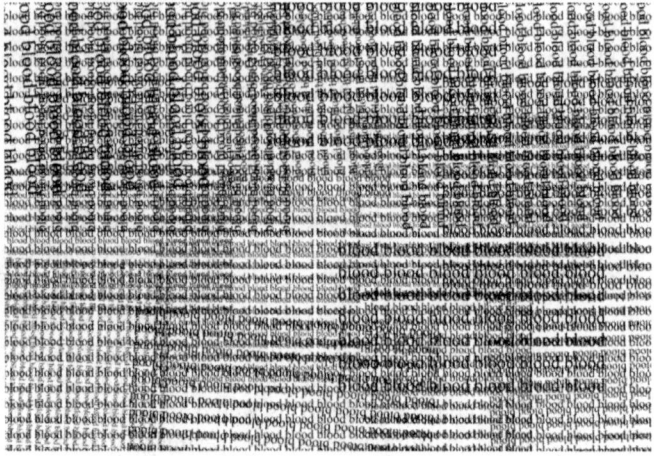

I fear that at some point Syl will become repulsed by her own body, its piercing alarms, the bumps in odd places, the sense of being patched together. A different repulsion than typical pubescent disgust. That she will find no love there. One item on the infinite list of concerns I have no answers for. I can imagine offering her an example she will not appreciate, a bodily earthly metaphor: James Turrell's *Roden Crater,* a preexisting geographical monument in Arizona's Painted Desert excavated into an experiential installation. Stone light shadow. My wish for Syl is Turrell's wish for his unfinished masterwork: "to set up a situation to which I take you and let you see. It becomes your experience."[10]

Rather than things being born, they are created. Björk creates and creates and creates, down to the transformative pronunciation of individual words. "Twist your head around," she sings, and in my ear it implodes, morphs, flexes, becomes, "Trust yr head around," the language body in buoyant freefall, both itself

---

10 James Turrell, *Roden Crater,* https://rodencrater.com/about/. I confess I am not exactly sure how this rather Situationist impulse might apply to the experiencing of one's own body. A purely intuitive observation.

and its other, a twisted bit of disjecta membra trusting it will land soundly —

trust yr, twist yr, create yr head. It is, after all, your head.

II

Polemic

On Diabetes Twitter users troll Big Pharma. "$800 a month for my insulin," writes one. "More than my rent. Might have to start rationing."

Chronic conditions a $iphon.

Diabetes mellitus, derived from the Greek word *diabētēs,* meaning siphon — to pass through — & the Latin *mellitus,* meaning honeyed, sweet. Sweet the excess sugar in the blood, the urine, the sugared urine noted in the literature of the ancient Greeks, Chinese, Egyptians, Indians, Persians.

To be one who sipped urine. A water taster.

The first known suspected description of diabetes can be found in the Ebers Papyrus, c. the sixteenth century BCE, Egypt. The Wikipedia entry for diabetes notes how a physician from these early years of diagnosis described the patient's urine as being too *asha,* too plentiful, too often, & prescribes "a measuring glass filled with Water from the Bird pond Elderberry, Fibres of the asit plant, Fresh Milk, Beer-Swill, Flower of the Cucumber, & Green Dates."

Other remedies included rectal injections of olive oil, honey, sweet beer, sea salt, & seeds of the wonderfruit.

Urine sweet enough to attract ants & flies.

The pissing evil.

In old China, "the wasting thirst."

Ancient Grecian doctors prescribed exercise, preferably on horseback to help alleviate urination.

Areteaus of Cappadocia, writing in the second century, describes the disease as "a melting down of the flesh & limbs into urine."

"Life," with the condition, he wrote, "is short, disgusting, & painful."[1]

Into the early twentieth century common treatments included bleeding & opium. Some patients were directed to eat as much as possible to replace the nutrients being lost through excessive urination. Others were instructed to consume large quantities of sugar. Those patients died quickly.

The starvation (rationing) diet proved more successful at extending lifespan. This method often involved physically restraining those incapable of controlling their urges. Who got hungry.

From rationing food to rationing insulin.

Kevin's Law grants pharmacies the ability to distribute emergency supplies to patients in situations where prescriptions are unable to be refilled, such as during national holidays.

---

1   Richard Barnett, "Diabetes," *The Lancet* 375, no. 9710 (2010): 191.

It is named after Kevin Houdeshell, who passed away in 2014 at age 36. He died alone in his apartment of diabetic ketoacidosis, after being denied access to insulin when his prescription expired over the New Year's holiday. He had been insulin rationing in the weeks leading up to his death.[2]

He lived in Ohio.

On land that belonged to the Iroquois nation.

In the US, native populations are the demographic most struck by diabetes. Nearly 15% of First Nation persons are dx with the condition.

Roughly 12% of Black Americans & those of Latinx birth.

Whites, at 7%, are at the bottom of the list.[3]

Cases of t1d account for approximately 5% of all diagnoses of diabetes.

Research will tell you the factors that contribute to certain demographics' higher rates of diabetes are "complicated," but they are not. Simply: The systems constructed around diabetes care are, like nearly every other (im)measurable system based in the relationship between governance & corporate greed, reliant on the injustices & inequities necessary to drive capitalism.

In 1922 the first patient was treated using a purified hormonal extract obtained from the pancreas of a cow. This extract was termed insulin.

---

2 Joseph Fink, "Kevin's Law Makes 72-hour Supply of More Medication Available to Patients," *Pharmacy Times* 87, no. 10 (2021): 54. Fewer than half of US states have adopted this legislation.

3 Centers for Disease Control & Prevention, "National Diabetes Statistics Report" (2020), 4, https://www.cdc.gov/diabetes/pdfs/data/statistics/national-diabetes-statistics-report.pdf.

Frederick Banting, Charles Best, & JJR McLeod, upon being granted the patent for their development of insulin, transferred the patent to the University of Toronto for the token fee of $1.00, in hope that public access to the formula would discourage a pharmaceutical monopoly & promote fair access for all.

The arrangement was lauded & deemed a step forward in medical ethics.

A century later, in 2022, a vial of insulin retailed for an average of $300.

As a lowball estimate, a typical t1d adult might go through 2-3 vials per month.

$1.00. Capitalism is a killer.

Exemplum

1.

Stock market a graph of rich. People feelings. My mind sad. Slow. Depression-era crash. Frank Ocean on headphones. Losing self-control.

Caffeine fatigue. Jittery fingers. Morning insulin. Won't get in the syringe. Prescription list. Stuck on the fridge. I ring the pharmacy. To fix their misreads.

Control-G their ability. To scan a script. The t1d mixtape. Sampled spastically. It freaks me out. This baring. Of dependency

on the supply chains & systems of the capitalist monarchy. What if. We go to war with China. The power goes out. I can't think too long.

If I couldn't get my hands on. A steady stockpile. Of the hormone that keeps. No space. To ruminate just. Get through the day.

Get through the Golden. Age of Dread. Kierkegaard: "Unhappiness never lies in [the] lack of control over external conditions."[1]

Point taken, but damn. Pattern recognition. Search-bar species. Look at me. Whine & pout. In the house where I live. Out the fantasy.

That I can just live. & now in the spare I've got Death as a renter. Always in his room. Tracking the financial sector.

2.

How to write this future. Futureless. Or further. Jump dimensions. À la Rick & Morty. Locate Syl's other versions. Ones not prone to hypertension.

Stroke. Nephropathy. Neuropathy. Of the gut. Face sex the ulcered foot. The butt & but. Ellipses trailing every acrid piss. The but

of decision. Warping future. Kidney function. Warping. Retina. Cataract fabricators. Fabric irritating skin. Flamed w/ infection. Deflect

the pregnant tendency. To stillbirth. Miscarry. Toward gum plaque & the macrovascular. Heart accumulating. Arterial plaque. How to write.

This futureless future. Irrelevant. How to macro. Your heart spectrum. Uncomplicate. The dis-eased. Moment. -um. Death of course is.

A complication. A question. Or radiance. Too often a received dictum. Then & then. How to grow yourself. Into a gentle

---

1 Søren Kierkegaard, *The Essential Kierkegaard,* ed. and trans. Howard Hong and Edna Hong (Princeton: Princeton University Press, 2000), 188.

plant or. A room to house. Survival. Vined to disproportionate. Dimensions. How to take care & be. Care. How.

Dancing the Machine: On Robyn's "Fembot"

1.

I started listening to Robyn riding shotgun in my friend's car.

I started dancing to Robyn on the blistering summer concrete of a loading dock.

Dancing on my own.

I started loving Robyn while riding my bike with headphones on, chewing gum.

Robyn like a tough leaf, a punch in the face, a backward somersault. Robyn like a plate of nachos heaped with salsa, chicken, and extra salt.

I started singing to Robyn on my living room carpet, pure workout-video vibe.

Pure cardiac cathartic co-lung collapse.

I started watching Robyn videos. Robyn on tour. Robyn in a dark room. Robyn in a warehouse, dancing ecstatically while imploring some nameless someone to break up with their girlfriend.

"Call Your Girlfriend" is one of my favorite music videos. Robyn in platform trainers, confetti leggings and a shag-carpet shirt dancing her ass off while a camera follows her around a vast, emptied interior. She's singing such sad, defiant, hopefully hopeless lyrics and at the same time having so much *fun*. The joy in what can never be. It's all giddy heartbreak, a blood clot in the aorta that dissolves into streamers and strobe lights.

That moment around the three-minute mark when she musses her perfectly styled hair: the practiced cracked veneer.

Robyn the touchable untouchable.

My Robyn is the Robyn of *Body Talk*. The triad, the spliced together pieces. *Pt. 1, Pt. 2*, the culminating full-length. The gentle acoustic version of "Hang With Me," the Swedish folk song "Jag Vet En Degli Rosa" pressed up against the propulsive synthetics of "Dancing on My Own," of "Fembot."

I started loving Robyn while working a recycling gig that required latex gloves to be stretched over my fingers. Fingering metals, plastics, organic composts. Wondering at how the world feels different through synthetic skin.

2.

"Fembot" has never been one of my favorite Robyn tracks, but I am obsessed with it, for the way it positions itself as a machine body.

Robyn: "I've got some news for you / Fembots have feelings too."

Donna Haraway: "A cyborg body is not innocent; it was not born in a garden; it does not seek unitary identity and so generate antagonistic dualisms without end (or until the world ends); it takes irony for granted."[1]

While a fembot, by definition, is not cyborg but rather android, the pop star declaring herself a fembot forces the reading toward cyborg by layering human performer upon roboticized performance. Flesh complicates. Here the feminine robot, a machine first introduced into popular culture by men and who was purposed for male-driven pleasure and weaponization, deviates; while the container may be a male byproduct, the intent, the driver, no longer is.

In this way "Fembot" skews meta as a commentary on Robyn's career within the music industry. An industry-generated pop prodigy, in the mid-1990s she released her first single at the age of fifteen, gained immediate fame, then endured a decade of her record label attempting to dictate the shape and sound of her career. A familiar story. One Robyn was determined to rewrite. In the early 2000s she left her label and founded Konichiwa Records. In 2005 she released *Robyn,* which *The New York Times* described as "swaggering, clever." She considers *Robyn* her first album.

Then in 2010 came the triptych. Three albums presented as a singular project, that spoke to each other, cross-referenced one other, held up on their own but didn't fully function without their adjacents. The album in cyborg form: *Body Talk.*

3.

Dance music is not innocent. It takes irony for granted. Robyn is a dance/pop musician, and for all the earnestness and tales of

---

[1] Donna J. Haraway, "A Cyborg Manifesto," in *Manifestly Haraway* (Minneapolis: University of Minnesota Press, 2016), 65.

failed love her songs project, she is acutely aware of the flipside of her genre's emotionality, of the need to "let the funny in," as the protagonist of Sheila Heti's novel *How Should a Person Be?* might say. Dance music is as ridiculous as it is austere, as goofy as it is cathartic, is both play and purpose rolled tight like good sushi served with a wasabi beat that lights you up, elevates your pulse.

Body Talk is to dance. Body Talk as a phrase also references the idea of body language, the work of communication our bodies do. While googling, I stumbled across a series of Body Talk worksheets for kids that demonstrate the "rules" of non-verbal talk:

> Tone of voice — Sounding interested/bored/excited etc.
> Posture — Standing straight
> Hygiene — Showering and putting on clean clothes
> Voice volume — Not too loud and not too low
> Facial expression — Happy/sad/excited etc.

That nonverbal modes of communication dominate our interactions is old chatter, but seeing these instructive lists got me thinking about authenticity and how much of our body talk is dictated by the strictures we are fit with as children. Are these instructions, in a way, meant to be read as how a person should be? The ableism present here disturbs; the assumption that a person must be able to perform these actions to be deemed acceptable, to present properly. These worksheets read like instructions for how to build a society of robots, replicants that do as they are told, that perform behavior within the boundaries of their written code. They march in lines down institutionalized hallways while the cyborg dances through the hybrid forest, testing the boundaries of her forms, the pieces she must cobble into the creature that is herself.

Body Talk may also (probably not intentionally) reference the holistic healing system of the same name. Founded by John

Veltheim in the late 1990s, the BodyTalk System blends yoga, acupuncture, and kinesiology into a "non-invasive method" of helping the body rid itself of stress.[2] Kinesiology is the scientific study of bodily movement, acupuncture seeks healing by addressing the energy fields in and around the body, yoga melds movement and energy into a sort of slow dance that spills open the spirit — again, dance intervenes, dance shakes self into selflessness, dance pains, injures, heals, dance is head work, heart work, dance is a body misunderstanding itself in the discovery of all it is not.

I do not know what Robyn's intentions were in naming these albums *Body Talk,* but I would guess them to fall somewhere along the lines of: let's talk it out with dance. Let's heal and love and cry to the strobing beats. Become one with the machine. Let's body up. Pump our fists, shake our heads. Get mechanized. Let the funny in.

4.

Maybe there is irony in calling "Fembot" one of Robyn's most human songs. The track sounds like a revved-up hard drive, stuttering synth and electronic beats, a looped moan that might have been ripped from the woofers of a sexbot. And layered atop the machined instrumentals Robyn's voice lands, crunchy with auto-tune, singing lyrics that sound like a list of computer part references, a list of ridiculous body and sex puns, totally over the top and perfectly situated in their don't-give-a-shit attitude. We see the robot attempting language and failing, wanting to feel and failing. We see the robot failing, falling apart, crashing, rebooting. How many times can a system reboot?

It is like a writing prompt: the freedom found in the restrictions of form. And form demands failure, in the way that reveals

---

2   Celeste Chong, "History of the BodyTalk System," *The Inside Job,* December 16, 2019, https://theinsidejob.sg/history-of-bodytalk-system.

failure as its own type of success. In adopting the fembot body Robyn wriggles into a space where she can talk about difficult shit in a way that is playful, absurd. Critics of the song are quick to point to the lyrics as its weak link. I would say they fail successfully. They embrace the ironies of womanhood — the championing of domestication, sexualization, optimization — via the imagery of an overtaxed machine frying its own motherboard.

5.

"Fembot" was born out of Robyn's consideration of her own aging body (as she turned thirty), and the power of the female body to bear children. To replicate. To reproduce. As she said in an interview with *Stereogum:* "People expect things of you, like kids and like marriage, and I found myself just thinking of that a lot while making this record, so ['Fembot'] is about that in a way, but it's also fun. I'm playing around with the concept of being a woman, and what it means to physically be able to carry kids, but at the same time that's not always what you see yourself as."[3]

If the natural female body might be read as a machine, then what of the female body that is also literally part machine? Do the expectations change? Does the mechanized cyborg form allow for a woman to operate more freely outside of the expectations of marriage, kids, job, appearance?

In a passage discussing Donna Haraway's "A Cyborg Manifesto," Jia Tolentino takes up the idea of the cyborg as a model for women to move beyond the compliant behavior of the expected, "optimized" life: "[The cyborg] would understand that the terms of her life had always been artificial. She would — and what an

---

[3] Jessica. "Progress Report: Robyn," *Stereogum,* March 10, 2010, https://www.stereogum.com/292372/progress-report-robyn/interviews/progress-report/.

incredible possibility! — feel no respect whatsoever for the rules by which her life played out."[4]

Robyn, in her playful questioning, is joyfully entrenched in that disrespect. She embodies the punk-bot. The pop-bot. The electro-punkpop cybernetic. The gynoid turned goofy revolutionary. The human born of mass production, the factory baby unfit to fulfill the cycle.

6.

Yet from the vantage of the cyborg herself, or of the cyborg's caretakers, I imagine this vision of the cyborg as some "oppositional, utopian" being falls somewhat flat. At least it does for me. Managing the cyborg body is difficult; the upkeep and servicing are constant. The machine is not autonomous.

There is a line in "Fembot," a refrain intoned in a voice pitched low and auto-tuned to the point of distortion, to where it nearly blends into the squelchy electronics of the track: "Once you've gone tech, you ain't never going back." I had always heard this line for what it is, a silly pun on a bit of sexual innuendo. Yet now, listening to the track in the shadow of new circumstance, this line caught me off guard — the hard truth of it. Because, for my daughter, her reality is wrapped up in this pun. Diagnosed with t1d at the age of thirteen months, she will never know what it is like to live in a body not reliant on machines. "Going tech" is not simply the exploration of an other; the other, for her, is necessity. There is no back to go to.

I suppose you can read the line as a woman claiming ownership of her body, "tech" synonymous with power, choice, resistance. But.

---

[4] Jia Tolentino, "Always Be Optimizing," in *Trick Mirror* (New York: Random House, 2019), 92.

What about those for whom the phrase reads literally? I would guess it was not Robyn's intention to signal toward disability, but it is there. An undercurrent of misconstruction. That line squeezes a lot of the fun out of the song for me.

Maybe it's my mood today. It just hurts, when it catches you from the side, or in a stupid song hook, the fact that my daughter will have to carry her disability through this life. Will have to carry it, ultimately, alone. That however much I or her mother or the algorithms have her back, she's the one wearing the machines.

7.

Don't get me wrong. I still love Robyn. It's just more complicated than it used to be.

Dancing on my own just doesn't cut it.

Parenthood turns you into a robot of sorts, the rote, repetitive behaviors, change this, wipe that, pick up this, fold that, eat sleep slobber piss. Servile. Childcare as a fixed form one moves, stretches, flexes within.

But eventually the form cracks. Things don't go the way they are supposed to. For us it happened earlier than for most, later than for the brave few. My daughter was dying. The technology gave her back to us.

There is an aloneness in Robyn's fembot that doesn't resonate with me. Maybe it is the irony of illegitimacy, that a fembot/cyborg might actualize selfhood in being unfaithful to her origins, as Haraway says. The illegitimacy that renders the father inessential.

The expectation in donning the fembot armor seems to be that men won't change. That they are brutish bastards, always have been, always will be. I don't know that I can argue with that.

Only that, in being present to my daughter's needs, her tenuous cyborg form demanding of every day a disciplined attention to the body and its mechanized appendages, I have changed.

In handling her synthetic parts I have seen her, see her, the human, physical her, in such focus. The slow removal of each device, working the bonded patch of insulin pump or CGM away from her form. The strange imprint left on her skin that looks like she either got branded or just had a piece of circuitry implanted beneath the surface of her. Picking leftover medical adhesive off her stomach, legs, arms, back. Taking stock of the constellation of puncture scars on her belly and thighs. The way she grimaces, shakes her head, cries out — her hand squeezing my finger against the dull pop each device makes at the moment of injection.

Our routine of maintenance and replenishment. Disobedient dances we don't dance on our own.

Exemplum

3.

On the table the new. Arrival. Syl's CGM. Continuous. Glucose. Monitor. Sixteen months old. Three months post-diagnosis. I spend an hour browsing

YouTube. Tutorials. Prepping to fit my daughter with her first. Machine assistance. Everyone online. Claims it's a game. Changer. The name of the game:

How To Die Slower. I hate the idea. This electric device adhered to her. A thin metal filament. Shot beneath the dermis. To socialize. With her interstitial fluids.

I grab the plastic applicator. Looks like Boba. Fett's bounty hunter ship. Kate cradles Syl. I tug her waistband low. Adhesive to the fatty. Lower

back. Press the orange button &. Syl howls. Flails. I see a trickle. Of blood beneath. Shit. No — in the YouTube comments, one user said a bleeder is.

A taker. Syl scratches at it. Shouts at it. An hour later she's forgotten it's there. Like a shark. Wears a sucker fish. I stare at it. Continuously. Wonder what this makes her.

4.

Rx Sonnet

acetone (urine) test strip ketostix
glucose blood VI test strips (Verio)
insulin glargine injection (Lantus)
100 UNIT/ML   insulin lispro

injection 100 UNIT MISC
(Humalog)   ONETOUCH DELICA LANCETS
33G   Continuous Blood Glucose
Receiver   B-D INS SYR HALF-UNIT

.3CC   god you mother-
                (PRECISION XTRA) KIT
0.3 (DEXCOM G6 RECEIVER)
Continuous Blood Glucose Transmit

alcohol blood swipe (G6) remover
glucagon rdna 1 MG SOLR

A Cyborg's Father

"Be really gentle this time," Syl says. She points her index finger and I place the spring-loaded lancet, set at its lowest setting, firmly upon her fingertip and press the button. She twitches, shivers. I milk a drop of blood, wipe it, milk another, let the test strip lap it up. "That wasn't so bad," she says, licking away the leftover traces of red.

To gently draw blood. In that phrase, fatherhood. To wound and wound in hope the pain will keep the child alive. To do so in a way the pain appears generous, a gift. *Here,* we say to Syl, *let us cut you open. Let us show you what is inside of you. Let us chart in blood the numerics of what has gone wrong. Let us say thank you. Let us cringe when you give thanks in return.*

I have little relationship with inflicted physical pain. My parents never laid a hand or belt or hard wooden object on me. Having my wisdom teeth removed is the most invasive surgery I've experienced. I have, amazingly, never been in a fight. Never punched, never been punched. At least not with the intention to *hurt*; like most kids my body got punched, pounded, tackled, slammed, tripped, tumbled, etc., and returned the favors in plenty. But those were games. To hurt one's small daughter, to of necessity again and again inflict pain upon her, to draw her blood into the air, that is real. I wonder, with each small stabbing, who is hurting more. On her end: the jolt of punished nerve endings. On mine: the hurt of hurting her. The self-laceration.

Anne Boyer, writing on pain, notes, "If pain were silent and hidden, there would be no incentive for its infliction. Pain, indeed, is a condition that creates excessive appearance. Pain is a fluorescent feeling."[1] In an attempt to feel what Syl feels, several months after her diagnosis I check my own blood sugar. Press lancet against fingertip and squeeze. Fuck it hurts. Fluorescence, yes. Incentive, no. I take retroactive stock: in the first three months post-dx we had pricked her finger five, six, seven times a day: nearly five-hundred times. I am ill at the thought.

◊

Blood tells secrets. He scans the numbers of his lab results. His blood work. "All results are normal or nearly normal," reads the accompanying letter. Nearly normal. Define the range of normality. Total cholesterol: 148. White blood cells: 3.4. Most of the numbers mean nothing to him, their sense hidden behind abbreviations and acronyms. The "work" in blood work is the effort required to comprehend. He scans to the end of the document. A1c: 5.3. Not yet pre-diabetic. He feels exposed, revulsed, and momentarily full of health. Throwing the results in the recycling he sets off for the kitchen. He wants to eat something sweet and rich.

◊

Blood moves. Blood transports. Blood is not a fluid, it is connective tissue in the form of fluid. It is one thing in the guise of another. It is two things in one container. Blood brings food and disposes waste. Blood regulates. Blood clots. Blood is life. Blood is magic. Blood feeds the supernatural. Blood brother, venge-

---

[1] Anne Boyer, *The Undying* (New York: Picador, 2019), 215.

ance, baptism. The blood of guilt. Menstrual blood. Blood and wine. Blood and water. In cold blood. The blood of Christ.

My daughter lives closer to death's house than most. It has taken some time to get used to this. I will never get used to this. With every drawing of blood, with every drawing into sight what is meant to remain hidden, I am reminded. Blood red. The red of emergency. The state of emergency that composes every day. The sight of blood for some wipes the conscious mind out: they faint. Vasovagal syncope. This response is thought to be a primitive reflex born of self-preservation. If your body is bleeding profusely from a wound suffered in conflict, fainting would make you appear dead. If you look dead, it is less likely you will be killed. Fainting also forces the body to lay down, which forces blood toward vital organs such as the brain. I don't pass out at the sight of blood, fortunately. Nor does Syl. It is easy to forget, amidst the routine woundings, that we are flirting with the primitive self, the mimicry of death, the mind's refusal of the body's experience.

The devices Syl wears, her CGM and insulin pump, are meant to decrease the sense of perpetual emergency present in the condition. And they do, in that we are less often confronted with the sight of her blood. There is less poking and jabbing. There is relief in that. And yet their appearance is excessive. Despite being small technological wonders, they hulk, transfigure, announce. They signal pain: the brown stains of blood from the CGM's sharp insertion pop often leak into the adhesive fabric; the pump's small window through which you can view the cannula inserted into skin, see the pain site.

They signal difference, otherness. They are like flares driven into roadside gravel, sparking news that an accident lies ahead in the darkness.

Diabetes is called a silent disease. Silent because it hides, can be kept hidden. Glucose checks in bathroom stalls. Syringe needle stabs through shirts, under tables. Syl's grandfather, also a t1d, once described himself as a silence addict; he would do anything to keep his condition hidden, to maintain the appearance of normalcy, to present the illusion that everything was fine, as it should be. To this day he has a habit of disappearing from the room without a word, off to check numbers, to correct or treat.

As if his body's failings were a sin committed, a burden, an inconvenience to others.

Diabetes is also invisible in its ubiquitousness, in its cultural visibleness. The word gets tossed around, slapped into odd contexts, dropped as punchlines, used as shorthand for insensitive critiques. *Of course she has diabetes, look how fat she is. Or, You ate that whole quart of ice cream? You're so going to get diabetes.* There is a general sense that all diabetes is related to sugar, somehow. Beyond that the ignorance is profound. But it is an ignorance accompanied by a familiarity with the word, the idea. Everyone believes they know diabetes until they are confronted with the reality of it. The condition itself hides behind the mask of its name.

Something similar has occurred around the word *cyborg*. Cyborgs are everywhere. They sit next to us on the subway, they cut in line at the grocery to buy kombucha and jerky, they populate our pop-culture fantasies. Most cyborgs don't consider themselves cyborgs. They are patients. They are survivors. They are chronic. Their machinery is kept under cloth or buried beneath skin. Is internal. Or walks beside them. We like our cyborgs undercover, shadow citizens, moving below the surface of perception.

◊

He considers choice. What is choice in the kingdom of chronic illness? There is always choice, but the choices aren't always good. He opens the cabinet and takes stock of the piles of his daugh-

ter's medical supplies. Choice. She might one day decide to give up using the CGM and insulin pump, to exist as a human fully naked. Still, even without the wearable technology she will be reliant on man-made tools: syringe, glucometer, and always that synthetic fluid, one of the most expensive liquids in the US, insulin. The machinery of life is corporate medicine's con job: that it is not ok to die. That we must live whatever the cost. That we will pay any price. Medical cyborgs are stripped of the right to life, to simply live: for them there is a monthly fee, a rent on breath, a financial chokehold on existence. Insurance another type of death. For all the talk of good intentions, better quality of life, he hears in the chatter the riptide of profit. Big Pharma's blood draw. The bleed. Of course he would do anything to keep his daughter alive. Of course they will exploit his love for every available cent.

◊

In season 4 of the Netflix series *The Crown*, the episode "The Hereditary Principle" brings to light the British royal family's treatment of several developmentally disabled members of their clan: lock them away in an institution and never speak their names. Katherine Bowes-Lyon and Nerissa Bowes-Lyon. Who, though childlike, knew they were part of the royal family. Knew who their relatives were. The episode follows Princess Margaret's discovery of their existence as she confronts her own mental health struggles. Horrified, she confronts the Queen Mother, who informs the princess that public knowledge of Katherine and Nerissa's condition would "make people question the integrity of the bloodline." Would, in other words, render the royals human, an impermissible fallacy.

When your child develops a chronic medical condition, you feel guilty. You want to hide yourself away. Even when the doctors and nurses and educators and the DOC tell you it is not your fault, it is nobody's fault, you don't believe them. How could it not be? How could there not be some latent genetic trait linked back to you, the trigger of her condition mixed up in your blood?

That there is no good answer for what causes t1d exacerbates the doubt, implicates the parent. *Her condition must be hidden somewhere inside of me.* How to not think, I did this to her.

◊

Japan has a long history of hiding its disabled from public view. I lived in Tokyo for a time in the early 2000s and have no recollection of seeing disabled persons anywhere. On the street, the subway, in restaurants, the school where I worked: nowhere. The cultural shame attached to disability in Japan is palpable, to be avoided at all costs. Though disability visibility there has purportedly improved in recent decades, a simple statistic illustrates the continued emphasis on shutting out disabled voices. In the United States 26% of the adult population is reported to be living with some sort of disability. In Japan that number is 4.8%.

In 2016 Satoshi Uematsu climbed through a window of the Tsuki Yamayuri-en care facility for disabled persons in Sagamihara with a bag full of knives and began stabbing residents. A former employee of the facility, he killed nineteen people, injured twenty-five more.[2] While on his rampage Uematsu reportedly screamed, "All the handicapped should disappear!" repeatedly.

Uematsu didn't need to resort to murder to make the Tsuki Yamayuri-en residents disappear. They had already been disappeared. The disappearance of being placed in a long-term care facility by their families. And following the attack, the disappearance of the victims by the local police, who decided to not release the names and faces of the victims in order to "protect the families who may be worried about discrimination."[3]

---

[2] "Japanese Man Who Killed 19 Disabled People Sentenced to Death," *BBC News*, March 16, 2020, https://www.bbc.com/news/world-asia-51903289.

[3] Matthew Hernon, "Why Is Japan Still Biased against People with Disabilities?" Tokyo Weekender, July 11, 2017, https://www.tokyoweekender.

Nameless, faceless. Author Suzanne Kamata said of the response, "Not showing their names and faces is basically like denying them their humanity."[4] The irony of the police response, that their attempt to protect the families from discrimination resulted in a more direct and blatant discriminatory act. To not publicize a person's name because they are disabled is pure erasure. Is to stand in solidarity with the murderer and say, This life was not worth recognizing. *This life was a life that should not have been lived.*

As horrific as this act of mass killing was, the invisible blood spilled by the complicity of the police may be the more chilling and pervasive of the two crimes.[5]

◊

He tries to be as gentle as he can, but it is hard, when welling blood from beneath the skin, to be gentle. Syl cries out at the jab. "Shout it out," he says. "Shout as much as you need to." As if to say: be as angry as you need to be. Be as brazen as a brass band blaring down Main Street. He wants to gather her into his arms and hold her. He wants to make like it's no big deal. He wants to throw these tools out the window, let them clatter into the street, get crushed beneath truck tires. These tools that he clings to like life itself. The onus of the technology cocktail: magically advanced, coldly barbaric.

◊

---

com/art_and_culture/japanese-culture/why-is-japan-still-biased-against-people-with-disabilities/.

4   Ibid.

5   The Cyborg Jillian Weise's poem "Attack List," from her poetry collection *Cyborg Detective* (Rochester: BOA Editions, 2019), is a startling take on the erasure and fetishism of disabled persons. The poem is built from news headlines that refer to the "actual murders and rapes of disabled women, as reported, primarily, by media outside the United States." A bullhorn of abuse coupled with a silence heard acutely by the disabled living inside US borders.

A CYBORG'S FATHER

Visibility is the radical act. To wear one's machinery out loud. To not be silent in the difficulty.

To be radical is difficult. Especially when the task is unasked for. What of the child who just wants to blend in? Who wants only to be invisible. The unwilling dissident. The chosen one. The child who lives like spilled blood, bright red dark red, the visible emergency of living flown like a flag in gusting wind, a raised banner that those who simply exist trudge beneath, oblivious.

Exemplum

5.

What is god in the light. Of diagnosis. What is god in the light. Of chronic illness. What is light. If light is god's trick. What is god in light.

Of what god isn't. What is god if god. Is a word. What's a word but a sandwich. Board. What is bread if your body. Rejects bread. If you break

bread and your body rejects. God. What is god if your body. Breaks with god. What is god in light. Of molecules. What is god if beyond. Assertion.

What is god if every single person shoves god. In their back pocket. Waits for the ringtone. What is god if you purchase. A ringtone.

What is god if. Infinite metaphor. Limitless value. Immanent Hasselhoff. What if god is just. The asshole you work for. Who won't give you leave to care.

A CYBORG'S FATHER

For your sick girl. What is god in light. Of crisis. What if it is god. Who designed the crisis. What if god is. The architect. Of your panic.

What is god if not. A form of queerness. A bright. Coded hunger. What is god but the self. You are taught to fear. What is god but the club.

Exit to the rear. What is god if not the beat. If not Black. Thought in a cypher. Untouchable syllables. Cyclone's eye. What is god if not killing.

Excitebike on NES Classic. Level up you bastards. What is god but a hole. In a hole. Donut-holed. That you swallow whole.

Hate yourself. What is god if you're the reason. Syl got ill. What is god if god. Negates control. If god is what. Just unfolds. Origami. The truth à la Lizzo.

What is god when you are part. Electronic. What is god when you trust. Algorithmic. Formulas to keep you. More than you trust. God.

What is god but a trauma anthology. A drama. Poetic history. What if your holy book is missing. Page 3. What is god when your phone.

Is your body. When an app. Is your body. Extended harmonic. What is god if god. Is histrionic. What is a tantrum. If the tantrum is god.

What is god if not your two-year-old. Throwing a fit. About what YouTube to watch. A machine assist. To switch out her machine with less drama.

Failure. What is god if the chronic. Is a form of death. Is god an extension of your credit. Card wealth. What is god when you are short.

On the ecstatic. When the problem of just living. Turns problematic. What is god if not a failed. Organ. What is an organ if not. A god's wail.

Making Visibility: Naomi Wu

The self-proclaimed SexyCyborg has breast implants
that light up when she wears a special corset. See her strut
heels and bikini top through the streets of Shenzhen, a modified
drone recording 360° of her journey in split
screen. "Just me in cute outfits when I'm not in my workshop,"
touts her Insta. See her YouTube channel, Wu in coveralls
tinkering at her workbench, 3D printing wearable
tech, hacking her new electric bubble trike. Body mods
make perfect sense to Wu, who sees her own form
as an enclosure, a machine that might perform its job
better with a few updates. "You have to give the computer
what it wants," she says. Wu envisions algorithms
on video platforms that give preference
to attractiveness. Naomi wants to be on top
of search results. Naomi wants to sell body part
upgrades. See Wu outside a maker conference in China,
strapped in a disruptive bra, protesting the casual
lack of women in the speaker and vendor lineup. See Wu brave
authoritarian arrest. See Naomi open
source herself as a model for all machine-laced
humans. "Not a model," touts her Insta. Disobedient
hardware. She designed and built that corset.

The self-proclaimed SexyCyborg has breast implants[1]

[1] The choice was between breast implants and leg extensions. Having one's femurs cut in half and lengthened with a metal insert seemed rather too invasive to Naomi Wu. She felt the extra inches of height weren't worth it. She could wear higher heels.

And not just any implants. Implants of such volume that, when coupled with the extreme heels she often sports on Instagram, give Wu the distinct impression of a top-heavy work of architecture whose construction you can't help but wonder at — how does it stay upright? (Lack of experience noted: I really have no idea how implants would feel (or breasts, for that matter). I have never really considered implants as a type of tool, which they certainly are. And I am, in relation to implants and body modification, intrigued by how fantasy and fetish might be viewed as a type of "add-on": that is, how tools like implants create an implicit cyborg state in a self via the projected fantasies of others (or of the self) onto the viewed/felt body.) Still, given the attention she receives from onlookers in the videos she posts of her public outings, plenty of people find her +++size breasts attractive, despite (because of?) their disproportion.

that light up[2] when she wears a special corset.[3] See her[4] strut

² When I first read about Wu's light-up breasts I came away with the impression that Wu had had lights implanted into her breasts. Lights that, when she donned a certain corset, were activated. Not so. The reality is decidedly more pedestrian, though the more ingenious for being so. Wu takes advantage of the translucency of human skin coupled with the refractive properties of her breast implants to create a lit-from-within effect using fiber-optic cable that runs from a retrofitted light source strapped to her back. The ends of the cable press against the outer underside of her breasts, shooting light through the clear, gelatinous silicone of the implants, giving the appearance that they are lit from within.[i] If you've ever pressed your palm against a flashlight bulb and been creeped out slash fascinated by the eerie red glow of your illuminated flesh, that's the "science" of the effect. The resulting outfit — illuminated body parts, thick black cables protruding from Wu like external arteries — is maximum cyberpunk. And total clickbait. On Wu's YouTube channel this video carries the tagline "Light-Emitting Boobies."

³ As evidenced by the light-emitting-boobies corset, Wu likes to make clothes. Or rather, she likes to modify pieces of clothing into wearable technology, or vice versa. She has outfitted a 3D printer with backpack straps to haul around the subways of Shenzhen, demonstrating 3D printing to any interested pas-

---

i M. Christian, "How SexyCyborg's Light Up Breast Implants Celebrate the Artificial," *Future of Sex,* March 11, 2020, https://futureofsex.net/augmentation/how-sexycyborgs-light-up-breast-implants-celebrate-the-artificial.

A CYBORG'S FATHER

sersby, part of her commitment to bridge the divide between DIY maker culture and the tech ignorance of the general populace. Other builds include LED-lit skirts, boots with projectors built in, and one of my favorites, the Wu Ying boot, which transforms a platform boot into a hacker's supply kit, each heel hiding a secret container modified to hold a USB keystroke counter, an ethernet cable, a wireless router, and lock picks[ii]: fashion built for espionage.

Wu's creations most often focus on how tech in clothing can interact with and augment the female body or take advantage of the unsung restrictions women often face in their consumer choices. The Wu Ying boots, for example, were born from the fact that women's clothing tends to not have pockets. Wu saw the platform boot, a popular height enhancer among young Chinese women, as an underutilized storage space.

I find myself considering my daughter in light of Wu's inventiveness. The t1d users of CGMs and insulin pumps are on the front lines of wearable tech, tech that immediately and significantly transforms the body, internally and externally. The external transformation is most promptly noticeable. On Syl's small body her CGM and insulin pump create significant bumps; there have been very few pieces of clothing we have found that truly hide either device. Complicating the matter is the need to rotate each device around various sites on the body — arms, stomach, legs, back — to maintain maximum effectiveness. For a consumer looking to minimize device visibility this seems the true challenge; clothing is so static in shape, generally — what might a moldable garment look like, one that doesn't adhere to ableist body structures but instead could be shaped and reshaped to the wearer's need and whim?

---

ii Michael Moran, "Sexy 'Human Cyborg' Plans to Give Mankind an Upgrade As She Shows Off Fiber Optic Glowing Boobs," *Daily Star,* April 17, 2020, https://www.dailystar.co.uk/news/latest-news/sexy-human-cyborg-plans-give-21821712.

MAKING VISIBILITY

Another option would be to refuse the idea that we need to hide such devices and instead celebrate their visibility. Wu's designs are geared toward helping us resee what comprises the body and how our bodies are both born and built. How might wearable tech be refashioned to make these life-giving devices focal points of celebration, rather than objects of bodily shame? Fashion model Lila Moss has embraced this approach. T1d since age eight, Moss unabashedly displays her CGM and insulin pump while walking the runway at high-profile fashion shows. The normalizing of the cyborg body by women like Wu and Moss is essential work for those who are cyborgs not of choice, but of necessity.

[4] Or don't see her. Naomi Wu is and is not Naomi Wu. Wu operates her SexyCyborg persona under a pseudonym. As visible as she appears, Wu takes great pains to protect her identity. Her identity, like her body, a purposeful construct. A made thing.

heels and bikini top through the streets of Shenzhen,[5] a modified

⁵ The city of Shenzhen comprises one of China's largest manufacturing hubs. Over the past fifty years the city has undergone a production and population explosion, spurred by Deng Xiaoping's 1979 "capitalism under communism" experiment. It seems to have worked. Today Shenzen boasts a GDP of over 350 million dollars a year, more than most small countries can claim. Deng's program brought an influx of government-driven incentive to do business in Shenzen, and with those economic incentives came the people: in the mid-1970s Shenzen's population was roughly 30,000; today it is a sprawling megalopolis of 12–18 million people (many Shenzen residents are undocumented immigrants, so census figures skew sketchy). That rate of expansion is nearly unfathomable. Imagine if New York City was a small college town in the '70s, and between then and now became the New York the world knows.

Shenzhen is currently attempting to recast its reputation from global manufacturing hub to a city of innovation. Naomi Wu is one of the more visible examples of Shenzhen's embrace of maker culture, the name given to the independent hackers, coders, tinkerers, and builders who aim to push tech and the ways we use it in new directions via a do-it-at-home methodology. The city's role as assembler for many of the world's biggest tech corporations has made it the ideal place for makers to thrive. As Wu observed, "I have middle-school-level shop/DIY skills, but I live in the most ideal hardware fabrication ecosystem in the world for these kinds of projects." If you have an idea and want to make it real, in Shenzhen, home to the Huaqiangbei electronics marketplace, one of the world's largest, the parts are available.

Though Shenzhen's factories produce many of America's most innovative products, most locals and those in surrounding rural communities can't afford to buy those products. This has given rise to a vibrant copycat economy. Think iPhones with peaches instead of apples as logos. Vendors selling Samsing instead of Samsung. Those hot-off-the-runway Bugo Hoss jeans. The ripped DVD of the latest blockbuster action flick, quality shoddy. Shenzhen popularized the term *shanzhai,* which originated as a derogatory term for knockoffs and pirated goods. *Shanzhai* culture, though seen in the west as rote imitation, is in fact centered around rapid and creative innovation. In their book *Blockchain Chicken Farm,* Xiaowei Wang discusses the work being done to reframe the perception of *shanzhai* as imitation. They cite the research done by David Li, founder of the Shenzhen Open Innovation Lab, and the scholar Silvia Lindtner, who propose the term "new *shanzhai."* Wang goes on to explain: "Part of the original *shanzhai* economy began with copying DVDs. Since copied DVDs couldn't be played by brand-name players, a whole set of products were created to support the copied DVDs. From there, a wildly creative ecosystem appeared." New *shanzhai,* then, builds off this adaptive ecosystem, which operates in direct opposition with notions of ownership and intellectual property prevalent in the West. It is open-source, amplified. Makers borrow, repurpose, co-opt, and remix each other's work. Innovation happens at breakneck speed. And, more importantly, it happens outside of corporate strongholds, who often build their products to discourage alterations to both hardware and software. *Shanzhai,* as Wang says, "holds the power to decolonize technology." It is our

A CYBORG'S FATHER

right, they argue, not only to use a device but to "collaboratively alter, change, and reclaim it."[iii]

The right to alter one's devices becomes especially relevant in the realm of medical tech. Diabetes care is a perfect example. Closed-loop insulin delivery systems, in which the user's CGM and insulin pump communicate with each other to make automated adjustments to basal insulin delivery to help prevent blood glucose highs and lows, have been viable for years, but most users remained years away from having access to these systems due to the incremental pace of FDA medical device approval. Rallying around the #WeAreNotWaiting hashtag, early innovators built an app that would use existing insulin-delivery technology to create a closed-loop system. Called Loop, the software has been refined over the past decade by the open-source community, drawing on the direct experiences of users to hone its features.

The obvious benefit of this technology is that it is free and available to anyone. And it works. It shows that when patients have a direct say in the creation of their care, they are able to replicate and at times surpass the quality of care that medtech corporations can provide, and can do so at a real-time pace, so that users don't have to wait years to access potentially life-altering or life-saving technology.

[iii] Xiaowei Wang, *Blockchain Chicken Farm* (New York: Farrar, Straus and Giroux, 2020), 132–33.

drone recording 360° of her journey in split
screen. "Just me in cute outfits when I'm not in my workshop,"
touts her Insta. See her YouTube channel, Wu in coveralls
tinkering at her workbench,[6] 3-D printing wearable

There are drawbacks to OpenAPSS (Open Artificial Pancreas Systems), however, especially if you, like most people, don't truly understand how things like your phone or computer work. Loop requires that its app be built from scratch on your phone. To use it you have to build an app. The instruction documentation Loop provides on its website is comprehensive, but — you have to build an app. For many this remains a major stumbling block, even if you already have access to all the necessary hardware (CGM, pump), which many don't (an entirely different and, honestly, more urgent issue). We considered trying Loop but opted against it after Syl got tapped to participate in a study for the closed-loop system in development by Omnipod. This was a huge stroke of luck, as the study allowed Syl nearly two-and-a-half years on this version of closed-loop before it became available for public use.

[6] Wu might be giving us a glimpse into our erotic futures. It's fascinating to watch her at work, piecing together her unique visions out of readily accessible hardware. Equally fascinating are the layers of self on display in her various social media. Wu's Instagram features a steady stream of her posing in revealing outfits, fully embracing the SexyCyborg persona. Her YouTube channel, on the other hand, is almost solely devoted to Naomi the maker: in her workshop, loose-fitting coveralls, a bandana wrapped around her head, the camera focused on the project rather than on her. Wu takes the artificial construct of the digital persona and pushes it into the realm of the physical: YouTube

tech, hacking her new electric bubble trike. Body mods make perfect sense to Wu, who sees her own form as an enclosure, a machine that might perform its job better with a few updates.[7] "You have to give the computer

Naomi is often building, literally printing physical objects that will enhance or spotlight her erotic being. As with her light-up breasts, the interaction between the natural and the artificial is being employed in ways that challenge what "attractive" means. With, say, the popularization of 3D printing, how will the ability to produce personalized body enhancements change the way we understand sexual and bodily augmentation? How will it radicalize and empower our personal pleasures?

[7] Wu is a transhumanist. Transhumanism advocates for the enhancement of the human condition using technology to augment one's functionality, mood, longevity, etc. Following a ruptured implant in one of her breasts, during the replacement surgery Wu had fiber optic cables inserted directly into her breasts, to further the effect of her light-emitting boobies project. While enhancements of this nature seem rather trivial, cosmetic surgery for Wu is not simply a matter of looking good, but a matter of expressing her sexuality and gender. She is a dee, a hyper-feminine lesbian for whom, she says, "cartoonish exaggeration of gender is very much part of the aesthetic." Hesitant to adopt further body mods such as magnets slipped under the skin (which, Wu points out, could be very useful in reconsidering how we wear our clothes and tech) or data storage implants until they have been proven safe for long-term use (heavy metal poisoning is a very real concern), Wu will continue to treat the

what it wants," she says. Wu envisions algorithms
on video platforms that give preference
to attractiveness.[8] Naomi wants to be on top

of search results.[9] Naomi wants to sell body part

body "like any other piece of hardware — subject to hacking and improvements until it suits our needs."[iv]

[8] Cosmetic surgery as body modification also plays a practical role for Wu. She recognizes that "surgery that makes you moderately more attractive has a higher return on investment than schooling that makes you moderately more competent."[v] Her vision of vision-based algorithms that push attractiveness to the top of search results sounds like the plot line to a movie but may just be darkly Darwinist enough to be prophetic. Her own videos are smart and fun; still, Wu would be the first to point out that it's the "sexy" in SexyCyborg that drives hits to her channel.

[9] It is delightfully subversive, the way she exploits human nature via unnatural methods to achieve her aims. Wu doesn't like the term feminist, but she fits perfectly into Haraway's feminist-grounded philosophy that a woman can use the patriarchal and capitalist structures imposed upon her gender as a form, an enclosure, within which to disrupt and sever the ties those structures bind around womanhood. At first glance Wu is not someone I would hold up as a role model for my daughter. You

---

iv Moran, "Sexy 'Human Cyborg' Plans to Give Mankind an Upgrade As She Shows Off Fiber Optic Glowing Boobs."
v   Ibid.

upgrades. See Wu outside a maker conference in China, strapped in a disruptive bra,[10] protesting the casual

lack of women in the speaker & vendor lineup.[11] See Wu brave

look and see skin, sex, followers followers followers. But at second and third and fourth glance she is exactly what I would wish for my daughter: a radical, protest-minded free-thinker who has purposefully and rationally carved out a space of her own.

[10] The "blinkini" is a nifty piece of tech-fashion. Composed of a series of small rectangular LED screens strapped across the chest and programmed by Wu to alternatingly flash opaque and transparent, the blinkini hides and reveals, teases and pleases. It is hard not to stare at, which is the point: worn in the context of the Shenzhen Maker Faire, the blinkini serves as a direct commentary on the Faire's male-centric take on maker culture. Wu wants to be included in the conversation. She demands it. The blinkini, an ingenious piece of wearable tech she pieced and soldered together, will make them look. Will make them stare.

[11] An active advocate for women in tech and involving girls in STEM, Wu pushes back because she has been on the receiving end of a constant stream of criticism and attempts to discredit her work. Even Dale Dougherty, the "godfather of the maker movement" and founder of Maker Media and publisher of *Make:* magazine, which have been credited with having laid the groundwork of what has become the modern maker movement, cast doubt on Naomi's status as a legit maker, tweeting, "Naomi is a persona, not a real person. She is several or many people."

authoritarian arrest.[12] See Naomi open

MAKING VISIBILITY

He followed this declaration by actively perpetuating the insinuation that Wu doesn't build her own tech in interviews, Twitter threads, and links to dank corners of the internet. Dougherty later recanted his statement, but his tweet remains the most high-profile example of the bullying Wu endures at the hands of the tech industry's machismo. It is no coincidence that Dougherty's barb came on the heels of Wu's very direct criticism of the Shenzhen Maker Faire's lack of female vendors and presenters: Maker Media is one of the Faire's main sponsors.

After bombastic online blowback against Dougherty's claims, Wu emerged from the spat on the cover of *Make:* and with a public apology from Dougherty himself. But the aftertaste of the episode lingers in the maker scene: the white, male, middle-age Western tech media mogul bullying the young independent Chinese female maker: a racist, misogynistic smear campaign.

[12] Wu's use of a pseudonym has a practical purpose: her lifestyle, her use of Western social media platforms, her protest and activist work, all fall out of line with what is considered in-bounds by China's authoritarian government and an aggressive cancel-culture present within China's tradition-oriented Netizens. She has made conscious choices to protect herself against the very real threat of detention, like not traveling abroad to participate in tech conferences, and having journalists sign agreements to

A CYBORG'S FATHER

keep certain aspects of her private life private. At the same time, Wu has written that "visibility is my superpower!" She exists in a space nearly incomprehensible to conceive for Westerners: a hypervisible, outspoken tech advocate and activist who also desires to keep a low profile, and expects those who profile her to listen to her desires.

Wu's relationship with Western journalism has been complicated and tense, largely, at least according to Wu, because journalists from Western countries are incapable of understanding the realities of living under authoritarian rule — where there are no set lines to be crossed, where you live day to day unsure if what you are doing is going to prick the skin of the wrong person — and see an individual's private spaces, sexuality, relationship status, etc. as open-access material, despite the subject's feelings. Take Wu's description of her online presence and how it might be perceived by Chinese authorities: "Every time you post something you have to guess. So, you wait. You wait for the sound of boots on the steps and a knock on the door in the night. If you have never been in that position, it's hard to describe. You try not to think about it."

There have been two instances of reporting in which Wu felt particularly threatened. The first occurred on the Netflix show *Patriot Act*, when Wu was included in a piece critical of Chinese leadership in China, without Wu's permission or factual verification. The show used a clip of Wu from a profile The Wall Street Journal had done of her years earlier, a clip of Wu discussing financial privacy that was taken completely, in Wu's words, "out of context." Taking such liberties in reporting is, for a resident of mainland China such as Wu, "insanely dangerous." It should

A CYBORG'S FATHER

be noted that while her actions do at times imply dissidence and certainly advocate for basic human rights, Wu has never directly criticized the Chinese government.

In 2018 *VICE* magazine sent a journalist to profile Wu. Naomi had the magazine sign her usual agreement that they would not disclose certain aspects of her life, those things that "any Chinese citizen would keep private," such as marital status, sexual orientation, family. According to Sarah Emerson, author of the article, after spending several days with Wu she reached out to ask her to respond to the Reddit theory that someone Wu is in a relationship with is behind her work. Emerson wrote: "I think the Reddit conspiracy theory is vicious, but since this profile is long and comprehensive, I'd love to highlight your opinions about prototype bias, gender expectations, and racism as they relate to the rumor. Let me know how that sounds, and what you're comfortable with." Emerson then claims that Wu wrote back calling the article a "hit piece" and demanded to see the profile before it was published, which runs against *VICE's* editorial policy. Wu also began writing confrontational tweets directed at *VICE* and Emerson, claiming that Emerson would be "throw[n] […] to the wolves" should the profile run.[vi] She even went so far as to dox members of the *VICE* editorial team, using her digital-projection boots to reveal their home addresses. *VICE* lashed back at this act and managed to get Wu's Patreon

---

vi Rebecca Watson, "Vice vs. Sexy Cyborg: How US Journalists Nearly Ruined a Chinese Maker," *Skepchick,* April 16, 2018, https://skepchick.org/2018/04/vice-vs-sexy-cyborg-us-journalists-nearly-ruined-chinese-maker.

account shut down, hamstringing a major source of revenue for the vlogger.

The profile that ran is glowing. Wu comes across as intelligent, ambitious, humble, complicated. As positive as the piece was, Wu obviously felt threatened by it. The problem, as she stated it, was the latent impression the article might give of influence by "Western hostile forces"; the Chinese state, at their whimsy, might decide that due to proximity or lifestyle choices that run against traditional cultural values a person is "foreign influenced." Such a designation could prove disastrous, dangerous even, for Wu.

So why would Wu agree to the profile in the first place? Visibility. Wu, at heart, is an activist. She understands that without visibility nothing will change. The tech scene will continue to ostracize and harass women, the PRC will continue to tolerate but not embrace the LGBTQ community, Western journalists will continue to sidestep her desires because they see her as a side column, something to gawk at then relegate to the archives. Wu is putting in the work to rewrite these narratives and doing so in difficult circumstances. Like she tweeted: "Visibility *is* the protest when you are a lesbian woman in Mainland China. When you are invisible they win, that's what everyone wants. To erase your inconvenient existence."

Or, as she wrote in an article on *Medium* that detailed her side of the *VICE* drama:

> Many Westerners are surprised that I'm so aggressive and think it's just me because it doesn't match what they expect — they don't realize it's perfectly normal for every Cantonese businesswoman I know. My grandma was a butcher and when toughs came to our little stall demanding protection money she chased them off with a cleaver — then came back and showed me how to swing it properly so I'd know when the stall was mine (slices not chops or it gets stuck in bone and you lose your weapon). I don't cry, I fight; I don't complain, I document; I don't wrap myself in victimhood and demand special privileges for it, I point out that I was targeted and insist I will work and study to succeed in spite of it — but I have every right to be angry. Anger drove me to help myself when no one else would. Anger — focused, controlled, directed appropriately and used productively can be as useful a tool as passion. I had passion, they gave me anger — now I use both like hammer and anvil. Without apology. If you teach young women that appropriate, focused, rational anger is "unladylike" you leave them with nothing but sadness — and tears don't get shit done.[vii]

[vii] Naomi Wu, "Shenzhen Tech Girl Naomi Wu, Part 3: Defunding, Deplatforming, and Detention," *Medium*, November 7, 2019, https://medium.com/@therealsexycyborg/shenzhen-tech-girl-naomi-wu-part-3-defunding-deplatforming-and-detention-140fed4b9554.

source herself as a model for all machine-laced humans. "Not a model," touts her Insta. Disobedient[13] hardware. She designed and built that corset.

MAKING VISIBILITY

[13] Not long after the *VICE* article was published, Naomi Wu was picked up by authorities near her residence in Shenzhen and detained. She was later released, shaken but undeterred. She continues to post as @SexyCyborg to YouTube, Instagram, and X (formerly Twitter). She is easier than ever to see.

III

Polemic

Fresh from the bath, Syl streaks through the kitchen. Shrieking hair a wet yellow. Tangle eyes devilish. Delight plump naked arms & legs pumping. Insulin pump on thigh. CGM on arm. Kate chasing.

Can a body be naked when rigged with electronics.

In a Facebook t1d group, one woman described how for the first time in years she had showered without her CGM or insulin pump. How incredible it felt. To shower completely naked. No rough plastic jutting from her skin. Just her body & the water. Her coarse, uninterrupted body.

Giggles float in from the living room. Kate wrestling Syl to the rug. Raspberry farts.

Dark outside. I am washing the dishes. Myself in the window, looking back.

Myself in the window like a fork.

Fished from the water & rinsed.

A CYBORG'S FATHER

Forked free of other possibility.

What is a body that, pressed against death's border, is allowed to remain a body.

A note written in cloud.

Oh, no you don't, I hear Kate say. A fresh round of thuds. Syl in a fit of belly laughs.

& for a few moments quiet, murmured conversation.

Into the kitchen Syl runs, face lifted, concern slanting her brow. She points to her leg, points to her pump. A flap of adhesive coming loose at the edge. She flicks at it, looks up.

I am falling apart, she says. *I am falling apart*

& I am down on the floor & she in my lap is whole is wholly herself what that is

I will never wholly know & oh

this something.

Unasked for, that has arrived.

At the inter

sectioning of my/our body

from hers. The inter

sanctioning of a body

with the horror of its other

with the beauty of its other

with the matter of its error

with the sectioning of its failure

with the searching for its other

with the error of its beauty

with the horror of its errors

with the matter of its intra

with the other of its matter

with the dark of its pleasure

with the pleasure of its failures

with the horror that they matter

Exemplum

1.

Uprooting Syl's CGM. Like a body part. Amputated. Plastic goofs skin. Like a bony part. Never studied art but. Electronics meets meat. Warholian —

more like Barney's *Cremaster*. Silver blended platinum polymer. Membrane infusion. The penetrating filament. Instrument. First apply the noxious. Adhesive

remover. Chemical yuck factor. Scratch & pick at. Her skin so. Soft her toddler whimpers. Yelps. As I tug the. Glue. Never have I felt more.

Cruel. Now cruelty's just something. I have to do. Stuck in the scene. No director, no jump cuts. Why's this shit so sticky. *Hold on,* I say. & rip.

A CYBORG'S FATHER

2.

!→→→→→→→→ " " →→→→→!!!↑↑↑!!!→→→→→→→→→→→→→→→→→
→ → → → → → → → → → → → → → → → → → " "
" →→!!→→→→→→→→→→→→→→→→ " " →→→→→→→→→→→→
" " " →→→→→→→→→→→→→→→→→→→→→→→→ " " " " "
" →→→→→!→!!!↑↑↑↑!!→→→→→→→→→→ " " " " " " "
" →→→→→→→→→→→→ " " " →→→→→→→→→→→→→→→→→→→
→→→→→→→→→→→→→→ →→→→→→→→→→→→→→→→→→→
→→→→→→→→→→→→→!!!→→→→! !!!!→→→→→→→→→→→ " " " "
" →→→→→→!!!↑↑↑↑!!!!→→→→→ " " " " ↓↓↓↓↓ " " →→→→→→ "
" " ↓↓ " →→→→→→→→→→→→→→→→→→→→→→ →→→→→→→→→
→→→→→→→→→→→→→→→→→→→→→→→→→→→→→→→→→!!!→→
→→→→→→→→→→→→→→→→→→→→→→→→→→→→→→→→→→→→
→→→→→→→→→→→→→→→ " →→→→→→→→→→→→→→→→→→→→
" " →→→→→→→→→→→→→→→→→→→→→→→ " " " " " →→→→
" →→→→→!!↑↑↑!!!→→→→→→→→→→→→ " " " " →→ " " " " " " " →→→→
→→→→→→→→→→→→→→→→→→→→→→→→→→→→→→→→→→→→
→→→→→→→→→→→→→→!!!→→→→→→→→→→→→→→→→→→ " "
" →→→→!!!!!↑↑!!→→→→→→→→ " " " " →→→→→→→→→→→→→→
→→→→→!!!→→→→→→→→→→!!→→→→→→→→→→→→→→→ " " →→→→→→→

SENSOR ERROR

→ → → → → → → !!!!!!!→ → !! → → → → → " " " ↓ ↓ ↓ "
" →→→→→→→→→→→→→→→→ " →→→→→→→→→→→→→
→→→→→→→→→→→→→→→→→!!→→→→→→→→→→! →→→→
→→→→→→→→→→→→→→→→→→→→→→!!!!→→→→ " " " " " "
" →→→→ →→→→→→!!→→→→→→→→→→→→→→!→→→→→→→→→→→→→→
→

SENSOR ERROR

" " →→→→→→ " " →→→→→→→→→→→→→→→→→→ " " ↓↓

SENSOR ERROR

144

EXEMPLUM

→ → → → → → → → !!! → → → → → → → → → → → → → → → → → !!!!! ↑ !!! → → → →
→ → → → !!!!! →
→ → → →

SENSOR ERROR

→ → → ↓

SENSOR ERROR

→

SENSOR ERROR
       ERRORE
       ERRURE
       FERRURE
       FERLURE
       FEIRLURE
       FEILURE
       FAILURE

Singing Creation:
On Mary Shelley's *Frankenstein*

Frankenstein is a flesh machine.

Frankenstein

A book is a kind of monster: plant-flesh repurposed into data storage. Information locker. Truth serum. Imagination tab.

It seems no coincidence that LSD is distributed on sheets of paper: to consume the flesh of the book is to hallucinate other realities.

We speak of text as having a "body." The body of a book is a built text, an archite(x)ture. I am interested in the built body.

I have been reading George Saunders's book about reading the short stories of the old Russian masters.[1] Tolstoy, Chekhov, Gogol. I have never been a fiction writer. The math of Saunders's

---

[1] George Saunders, *A Swim in a Pond in the Rain: In Which Four Russians Give a Master Class on Writing, Reading, and Life* (New York: Random House, 2021).

reading is impeccable. He builds equations out of narrative. Pattern recognition, charts, counting types of words and phrases. Emotional investment tricked out as a numbers game. A formula. I feel cynical about this. As if I wanted, what? The story as a magic talisman plucked from the gut of a sacrificial goat? The story as an impossibility? A divine gift? The magic of Saunders's book is that what is rather obvious feels, in his hands, magical. Making magic by unmagicking the magical. George Saunders was an engineer. The story, as he renders it, is an idea engineered with language, is language confusing the idea.

"I also became a poet… You are well acquainted with my failure."[2]

It has been decades since I last read Mary Shelley's *Frankenstein*. As I begin rereading, I am reminded of the purposeful structure of the novel, the nesting of story within story within story. The monster's tale told by Dr. Frankenstein; Dr. Frankenstein's tale told by the sailor Robert Walton, Walton's tale pieced together by the letters he sent his sister. *Matryoshka* dolls, set snuggly one inside the other.

I go to *Frankenstein* wanting tenderness. It is an odd place to look for tenderness, in the story of a pseudo-human built from the organs and limbs of the dead.

Syl has developed a fascination with death. She is three. She hasn't quite grasped the concept of dying yet. Her play is full of executions and resurrections, deaths sketched out in repetition. Here death is always followed by the promise of life. Rather than an end, it is a simple event from which the dead move on. Into life. Or into another death. Here the dead are animate: "They are all resting," Syl says, toys spread on the floor, "even the dead rat."

---

2   Mary Shelley, *Frankenstein or The Modern Prometheus* (Cambridge: MIT Press, 2017), 5.

Outside, in the first breaths of a storm: "A raindrop fell on my head," she says. "It died."

She was resurrected, this daughter. Taken from death's arms. Given life by the audacity of human invention. Reborn via electricity.

It is somewhat unclear exactly *how* Frankenstein animates his monster. Shock therapy? Incantation? What is clear is the unintended result of his painstaking efforts to create a beautiful individual: a being more hideous than his rich imagination could have conjured. Shelley's moral of creation: the more we strive toward beauty, the greater will be our failure in realizing beauty.

Her rendering of the monster is pure tenderness.

"I shall commit my thoughts to paper... but that is a poor medium for the communication of feeling."[3]

I am watching the band Big Thief perform their song "Mary" on The Current. The four of them sit in the studio, in a semicircle, three guitars and the drummer, instead of a kit, has in front of him another chair, this one loaded with a hodgepodge of items, plastic water bottles, plastic fruit, a flexible square of tile, of glass? Instead of drumsticks he looks to be holding cinnamon sticks. It is such a lovely song. The guitars pick and pluck their way through. The drummer taps and scratches at his odd cumulation, until, as singer Adrianne Lenker's voice falls away, he begins to stir them together, to knock them haphazardly from the chair. The apples and bananas and bottles bounce and thunk oddly on the hard floor. The tenderness of the song. The rattle and clutter of tenderness. And when the song ends they look at each other and laugh at that silly lovely experiment. A movement away from ease. A disruption that could have gone perfectly wrong.

---

3 Ibid., 6.

A CYBORG'S FATHER

The song organic, alive. In contrast: the artificiality of its making.

The person who lives with the aid of artificial parts is to be called what, then? We use the terms cyborg, transhuman, but they feel insufficient to capture the wonder, the blasphemous religiosity of (re)creation. Let us call them songs.

For some time I have wondered if *Frankenstein* was Shelley's reading, reenacting, of Wordsworth and Coleridge's *Lyrical Ballads*. As literary events the two works bear some striking resemblances, though those similarities take very different, even hidden, form. Most notably, both are concerned with the making and unmaking of a person.

Lyrical Ballads, as we read it today, was written by two people: William Wordsworth and Samuel Taylor Coleridge. However, when the collection of poems was first released, in 1798, this was not apparent. The book was published anonymously. There was no indication that the poems were written by more than one person; in fact, the book took textual and thematic pains to mislead the reader into believing "an Author" composed the volume, and in doing so birthed a fictionalized, fully realized, fully singular Poet. A curious experiment.

Then something happened. Two years after the initial release, in the year 1800, a second edition of *Lyrical Ballads* appeared containing a second volume of thirty-six additional poems. More importantly, a name accompanied the book: William Wordsworth. In the newly included Preface, Wordsworth mentions that a certain Friend composed several of the poems included therein. In that act sits a purposeful exploding of the notion of the singular "Author." And more, a large percentage of the newly included poems can be read as allegories of decreation: a collaborative act that goes awry; ruins; death; textual afterlives.

Something bothered Wordsworth about the existence of this Poet that was neither him nor Coleridge. Exactly what is impossible to say. He plainly saw something unnatural in this Poet's presence, something monstrous. He was determined to kill him off in the same way he created him: through poetry.

Frankenstein, published only twenty years after the first edition of *Lyrical Ballads,* in its plot charts a similar trajectory of making/unmaking as the collection of poems does over the course of its subsequent editions. Frankenstein, in collaborative conversation with the scholars and scientists who preceded him, through, importantly, books, stumbles upon a secret: how to give life. In striving to make a being, a work of art, of great beauty, he accidentally creates something he can't bear to look upon: a monster. The monster escapes and takes up a life of its own. Frankenstein sets out in pursuit of the monster, determined to erase its existence.

It is no accident that Shelley quotes "Rime of the Ancient Mariner" in the text of Frankenstein. That Shelley includes a passage from Wordsworth's "Tintern Abbey."

Frankenstein's monster and *Lyrical Ballads* 1798 are similar in their mode of construction. They are aggregates. The monster a collection of body parts. The book a collection of poems. Both are pieced together to create a thing more fantastical, more wondrous, than any of the individual parts could manage alone. A life.

Key to our belief is the unnamed ingredient. In the case of Frankenstein, we never learn the method by which he animates his experiment, outside the general clue that it might be tied to "electricity." That unknowing is necessary, so that the monster might breathe and walk. In the same way, it is the willful unnaming of the Author of *Lyrical Ballads* that allows its Poet to manifest into existence. They are both explorations/experiments of how language creates personhood. The built identity.

Our disabled populations continue to be beset by this perception. Of monstrousness. The abled in their eagerness to categorize assign words to those whose experience falls outside the typical. The disabled, like so many demographics, become other.

An othering which hovers between discrimination and potentiality. Full of space for the othered to engage in a radical disobedience. For neither the Poet of *Lyrical Ballads* nor Frankenstein's creation are ever able to be contained. They continue on. Language enables each to disrupt and exceed the limitations (death) their creators would place upon them. In seeking to kill their creations, both Frankenstein and Wordsworth only emphasize and perpetuate their existence. Or rather, the Poet and monster use the language that birthed them to disobey the desires of their makers.

"Of what a strange nature is knowledge!"[4]

says the monster as he slowly and secretly learns the "science of letters" from the small, impoverished family upon whose property he hides. The alphabetical technology that places a self outside the body, that divides and unites the human form from and with itself. A violent narrative rupturing that sutures us to the world. Awareness.

Syl's growing awareness of her machine parts has been fascinating to watch. As she has come into language, as she has begun to reckon the fact of the body with the knowing of the body, as she has come to understand the technology that is a part of her and separate from her.

Recently, after one of her insulin pump pods failed (accompanied by a viciously loud and piercing drone of an alarm — whenever I hear it I at first think it is inside my head, a tinnitus, an aural hallucination, it is of such an unreal frequency and tenacity), as

---

4   Ibid., 99.

I was applying a new pod to her thigh she tapped its plastic shell and said, as if speaking of an insect or an easily replaceable pet, "It's nice when they stay alive longer."

Andrea Brady: "Placed within the arrangement, the poetic subject gives up on the trope of 'strong responsibility' and transforms the fatalism of capitalist accumulation into song."[5]

Another term for cyborg is sympoiesis.[6]

The sympoiesis of family. Frankenstein's creature longs to merge with the small family he constantly observes, the blind elder father and his two grown children, to make himself visible, but is aware enough to realize *"I ought not to make the attempt until I had first become master of their language, which knowledge might enable me to make them overlook the deformity of my figure, for with this also the contrast perpetually presented to my eyes had made me acquainted."*[7] As his awareness sharpens, the idea of family begins to plague him. His memories, or lack thereof, gnaw at the edges of his consciousness.

"But where were my friends and relations? No father had watched my infant days, no mother had blessed me with smiles and caresses; or if they had, all my past life was now a blot, a blind vacancy in which I distinguished nothing. From my earliest remembrance I had been as I then was in height and proportion. I had never yet

---

5 Andrea Brady, "Alternative Arrangements," *FENCE*, https://fenceportal.org/alternative-arrangements/.
6 Donna J. Haraway, *Staying with the Trouble: Making Kin in the Chthulucene* (Durham: Duke University Press, 2016), 33. Haraway defines the word as "making-with." Other interpretations include "worldling-with" or "becoming-with." Haraway also points to M. Beth Dempter's earlier definition of the word, sympoiesis as "collectively-producing systems that do not have self-defined spatial or temporal boundaries. Information and control are distributed among components. The systems are evolutionary and have the potential for surprising change" (ibid.).
7 Shelley, *Frankenstein*, 92.

seen a being resembling me or who claimed any intercourse with me. What was I?"[8]

What was I. In Frankenstein's monster the built or machined body arrives into the world as an independent clause, unattached to lineage. It is of note that the creature's familial awareness comes on the heels, in the chronology of his education, of the political and economic realities of the society he sits apart from, the realization that ownership instills identity, and that he owns nothing. Not property, not lineage, not even a name. He has inherited nothing.

To the cyborg, the built body, the father is inessential.

And more, if we are to consider the man Frankenstein as the "father," the father is to be fled from. The father wants only to stamp out the othered body, to erase it. The father is to be resisted. The built body disobeys.

Feminist readings of *Frankenstein* explore the story's subversion of maternity and its depiction of patriarchal dominance. Here Victor Frankenstein becomes the true monster of the tale, in his bypassing of the natural order of procreation, in his refusal to give the creature a female companion. The father, the patriarchal system, that gives and takes away at whim. That determines the fate of those who are poorly born.

Mary Shelley surely saw herself in the form of Frankenstein's creation. How was a woman of her brilliance, whose take on everything from politics to romantic love was deemed radical in her time, to have existed in the world? How could she not have felt hunted, persecuted? The monster becomes both an idealization of the societally constructed body and the potentiality for dissent those constructs allow, as well as a lament. When a fer-

---

[8] Ibid., 100.

tile, imaginative mind finds home in such a form, to simply be oneself what choice is there but to flee?

Haraway writes, "Unlike the hopes of Frankestein's monster, the cyborg does not expect its father to save it through a restoration of the garden."[9] Shelley hurried the cyborg into the human imagination, but perhaps did not fully grasp the implications of this creature's existence. Haraway claims the cyborg has no origin story. Yet everything begins. Its origin, its exemplum, is here, in the fictions formed from the black aperture of personal apocalypse.

Matt Berninger, frontman of the band The National, found himself in the depths of a long depressive episode, convinced he would never write a song again. Deserted by ambition, by desire. By pleasure. Things he rediscovered in the text of *Frankenstein*, a book he grabbed randomly off the shelf in search of language, looking for words to "shake the tree and see what animals fall out,"[10] as he put it. Words that grew into the band's album *First Two Pages of Frankenstein*. Making living art out of shards from the past. Language a type of cyborg body, pieced together, living and dead at the same time, ordered and unruly, perfectly disobedient.

Frankenstein is a language machine.

I believe I have been mistaking reading for writing.

I sometimes look at Syl and wonder if she is a fiction. A depiction of life. A narrative being written in tandem with the forms, technologies, creatures that keep her alive. If she is a creative act. A Poet. A body in constant construction. Allison Bechdel,

---

9   Donna J. Haraway, "A Cyborg Manifesto," in *Manifestly Haraway* (Minneapolis: University of Minnesota Press, 2016), 9.
10 Matt Berninger, *Broken Record Podcast*, May 2, 2023, https://www.pushkin.fm/podcasts/broken-record/matt-berninger.

in her book *The Secret to Superhuman Strength,* writes, "I could see that the body, so disavowed by the patriarchy, was not something separate, or 'other.' Here, the other — including nature itself — was restored to the center."[11]

Frankenstein's monster first encounters beauty and pleasure while listening to the elderly blind father sing a song to his children. Amid the violent narratives of their lives, a simple music rises that returns the self to the center.

I often look at Syl and think, *song.*

---

11 Alison Bechdel, *The Secret to Superhuman Strength* (New York: Houghton Mifflin Harcourt, 2021), 92.

Exemplum

3.

Imagine the blood. A dancer. In the dark. (Blind Selma, dismantled Björk.) Folding into. Unfolding. Stone still. Molting. Form: shoulder, cheekbone, madcap. Percussive booby trap backslap. Filmic unspooling. Blue in the tooth. Ballad blurred.

+

Imagine the blood. A dancer tripping. On her own lip-sync. No taped stage. No mirrored referral. Dance an audience blind. Pitch lit photograph. Choreographic taxidermy. A voguesplashed singularity.

+

Image of the blood in sparse. Intervals. & faster. Till it strobes with the closure. Carried closer. Methodical. Visitant graced with plot. Points. A line traceable. Transfixes. Fixes into form the need. To receive. Each subsequent transmission. Live-streamed.

+

You participate. Consult & malinger. Envy & upend. Sag soft bottom into soft chair. Respond. Understand the expectation a communal expectation. Your own. Alarm blares. Square upon rectangle. Internal graph. High low. Diversion neuron. The diversion blood. Symptom it was a good day. All right & going. Well bad day. Handle your business. Damn. Notification. You panic. Watch the graph. Gotta gotta get. Up to get down. Your bodies the same. Bodies. Of points plotted. Numbers drop. Stomachs. Wait. Watch. Wait. Respond when. Prompted. You have to. You must.

4.

I want to be a dead thing. Syl says. Out for a walk. Riding Kate's back. Ripe country. Roadkill stink. *I want to be a dead thing* she says

again & laughs. She already is. Returned from the dead. Death like a cute shirt. Death a dermatitis. Infidel cells.

I want to be. A dead. Little comedian. Dante-esque. Who makes me. Shine & wince. How many times will she. Jump death. Grief.

Walks living. Amongst us when the death. Body lives out its death as life. We all already are. All things dead. Accumulating. Decay odor bad teeth.

Empty. Less judgements. Besmirched with dirt. Soft machines we. Climb the near hill. Free of stink the breeze. Vermillion.

Holly Herndon Creates a Life

Spawn is an artificial intelligence. An AI baby learning how to sound the world. How to snare and beatbox language into music's communal choir. For her 2019 album *PROTO,* Holly Herndon invited Spawn to collaborate with her across a series of tracks based in Southern choral music, the music of Herndon's youth. A music rooted in the very human act of singing together, of forming a community of song. Invited might be too strong a term — Herndon and her collaborator Mat Dryhurst built Spawn from scratch. They programmed and taught her, feeding her hour after hour of voice and sound samples. They learned how she learned. Herndon began singing simple and sensuous bits of language to her: *Aluminum cutlery can be flimsy. She wore warm, fleecy, woolen overalls. Alfalfa is healthy for you.*[1] Poetic fragments. Six months. A year. Eventually Spawn began to respond in ways distinctly her own. In ways that surprised.

What most strikes me about Herndon's approach to developing an AI system is how she considers machine life with such human

---

1 Holly Herndon (as told to Andy Beta), "Inside the World's First Mainstream Album Made With AI," *Vulture,* November 13, 2019, https://www.vulture.com/2019/11/holly-herndon-on-proto-an-album-made-with-ai.html.

A CYBORG'S FATHER

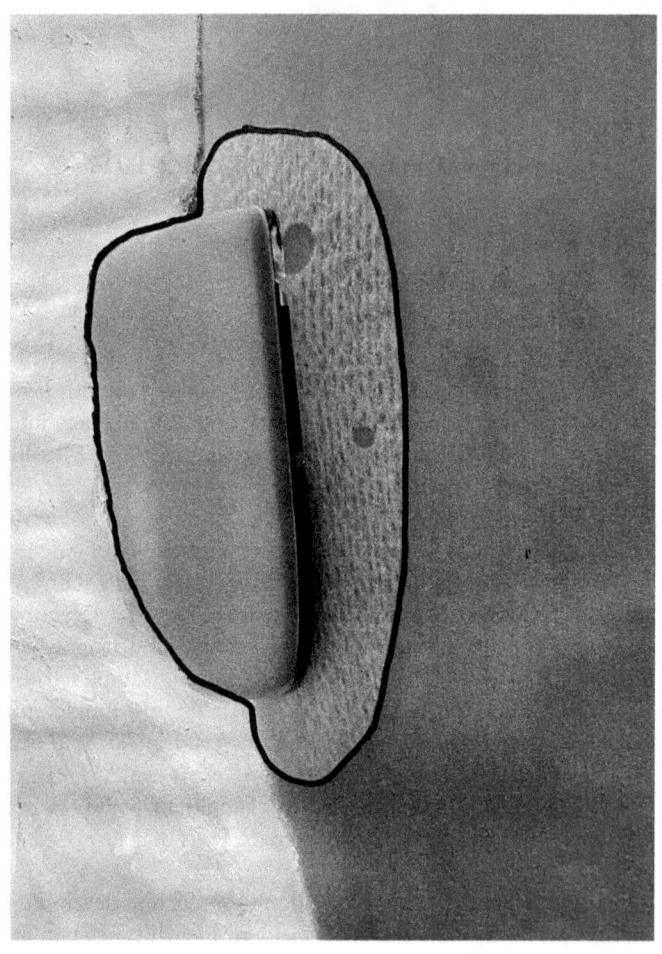

care. To her, Spawn is not simply a tool but very much a new being, one deeply influenced by the external stimuli and data sets it receives, one worthy of nurture, consideration, attention. Spawn, as she grows into her own voice, becomes a contributing member of the chorus, and Herndon is acutely aware that she is mothering Spawn into being. "What if the [way we raise her] could really have some sort of impact on how she grows up?"[2] Herndon muses, making space for Spawn at the human table.

Of her music, Herndon claims she is ever "trying to expand past the limitations of my physical body."[3] In this way she falls deftly in line with Haraway's vision of the cyborg. Why must our selves stop at the borders of our physicality? I am constantly reminded of this potentiality of human-/self-expansion with Syl whenever I consciously notice her CGM or pump: the ways in which they very literally expand her body beyond its borders, the way they expand her sense of self — how many people have we stopped to talk to simply because we noticed they also were wearing a CGM? One of Syl's sitters, also a t1d, gives her a "sensor-bump" every time they say goodbye. The visible machinery immediately propels Syl's body and self into a larger (and loving) community.

Amidst all the AI doomsayers, Herndon's vision of the algorithmic is the one I hope bears up. "There's a pervasive narrative of technology as dehumanizing," she says. "We stand in contrast to that. It's not like we want to run away; we're very much running towards it, but on our terms. Choosing to work with an ensemble of humans is part of our protocol. I don't want to live in a world in which humans are automated off stage. I want an AI to be raised to appreciate and interact with that beauty."[4] Again we see Haraway in Herndon's emphasis on choice and interaction.

---

[2] Holly Herndon, "Holly Herndon – Birthing PROTO," *YouTube,* September 10, 2019, https://www.youtube.com/watch?v=v_4UqpUmMkg.

[3] Ibid.

[4] Madison Bloom, "Holly Herndon Announces New Album PROTO," *Pitchfork,* March 11, 2019, https://pitchfork.com/news/holly-herndon-announces-new-album-proto-shares-video-watch.

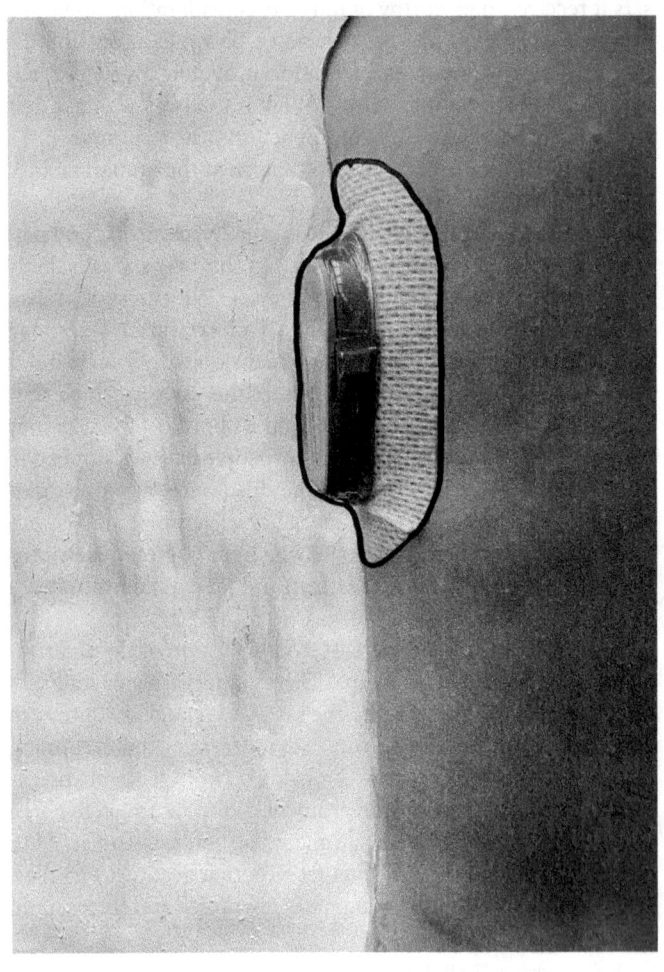

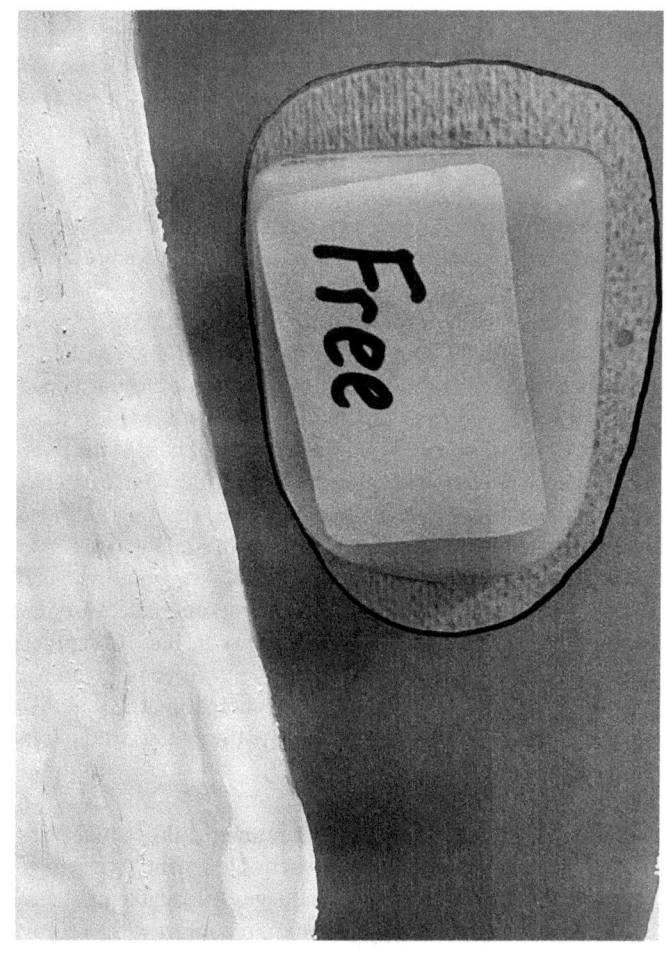

How we choose to interact. To inter-act. With whom and what we fuse our shapes, our selves.

Eve Kosofsky Sedgwick: "the open mesh of possibilities, gaps, overlaps, dissonances and resonances, lapses and excesses of meaning when the constituent elements of bodily, mental, or behavioral functioning aren't made (or *can't be* made) to signify monolithically."[5]

Syl's closed-loop insulin delivery system runs on a rudimentary type of AI and has already dramatically eased the administering of insulin, as well as improved her overall health and well-being. I can only imagine how these systems will continue to improve, as various modes of AI continue to fuse with one another in practically applicable ways. For a person with a chronic condition that requires dozens of small decisions a day (I can recall reading an article somewhere in which a t1d recorded the number of diabetes-related decisions made over the course of a day. They counted somewhere in the range of 280 separate decisions, a mind-numbing amount of mental and physical interruptions), having that mental burden lifted, even in part, would radically alter how one approached each meal, workout, date, workday, the timbre of a month, year, dare we say it, life. "Computers doing the heavy lifting […] really allows us to be more human together," Herndon says.[6] For certain cyborgs and those in their circles, AI might constitute a genuine pathway toward the freedom to just be.

Herndon describes Spawn as "an inhuman child." Child being metaphor for a nascent, incomprehensible technology. A figurative being, born of code. Of language. A readable existence. Spawn talks, sings, handclaps, creates, in concert with, a recog-

---

5   Eve Kosofsky Sedgwick, cited in Robert McRuer, *Crip Theory: Cultural Signs of Queerness and Disability* (New York: NYU Press, 2006), 156. Emphasis in original.
6   Herndon, "Holly Herndon – Birthing PROTO."

nizable music. An alien songcraft. "I would rather be a cyborg than a goddess,"[7] says Haraway. Spawn reflects a human condition: as we create increasingly humanized technology, we appear more alien to ourselves.

---

[7] Donna J. Haraway, "A Cyborg Manifesto," in *Manifestly Haraway* (Minneapolis: University of Minnesota Press, 2016), 68.

Exemplum

5.

In the voice of M, Syl's great aunt

I've had t1d for 52 years. Since 9th grade. Felt like I was getting the flu. Running laps in gym class I just about collapsed. My teacher, when she looked at me, gasped.

I was thirsty all the time. My urine was bubbly, foamy. The doctor sent me home with a bottle of pills. Those pills were so big. Horse pills. That was a Friday.

Mom was in California. Monday Dad took me to the hospital. It was packed. They put me on a stretcher in the hallway. Took a vial of blood four times a day.

Ed worked in the lab. I got to know him pretty well. Soon they moved me into a room with three other women. I didn't know what was happening.

My mom wasn't with me. Nothing was explained. My arms got so sore from the blood draws. I could hear Ed coming. His rattle.

He pushed a cart with all the vials of blood he had drawn. When I heard his cart, I would start to cry. I pulled the sheet over my head so he couldn't see me.

We still talked, though. Mom came home. I had been in the hospital for two weeks. I weighed 78 pounds. My arms were bruised black. They gave me an orange

& a syringe to practice injections. My parents wanted nothing to do with it. They never once picked up a syringe. They didn't try

learning & we weren't taught anything. I was given pee strips & told if the strip turned one color, I was doing things right. If it turned the other color.

I remember sitting at our dining room table. Dad sat beside me with a huge bowl of ice cream. He smiled at me & told me I couldn't have any. Thanks, Dad.

I took a job in California. I was 19. My commute involved two separate freeways. One morning when I got to work I didn't recall the drive at all. When I got to work I had a lot of candy with me.

My supervisor thought I was acting strange. She emptied my purse. Took my candy away. Called the paramedics. I woke up in the doctor's office.

No idea why I was there. I didn't know about checking my blood sugar. Only after I married R did I learn about glucometers. I was 26 years old.

I survived twelve years without checking my blood sugar. My first pregnancy I miscarried. The second time my doctor made me record my blood sugar constantly.

Nine months full of highs & lows. I loved being pregnant. It was stressful for R. E was born five weeks early. Healthy & perfect.

I first learned about my A1c when I got pregnant with T. I was told the number on this test should be 7 or lower. Mine was 14.

Because it was so high, they told me my baby was at high risk for all kinds of abnormalities. That it might never go home with me. A less-than-50%

chance of it being healthy. T was born two weeks early. Perfectly healthy. J was our third child. When he was 5 years old he began wetting the bed every night.

I didn't think too much about it. But one evening on a whim I checked his blood sugar. It was over 600. My heart dropped.

We did pretty good, J & I. Considering we didn't have an endocrinologist. We did the best we knew how. Our doctors would lecture us

about how terrible we were at managing our diabetes. There was no encouragement. I got up night after night to check his blood sugar.

Sometimes his numbers were so low. It was always scary for me. When J turned 19, he lost interest in taking care of himself.

He was hospitalized several times. For out-of-control blood sugar. One time for a terrible stomachache. X-rays revealed he had a hole in his stomach.

Without surgery he would have died. While hospitalized for that he developed a large sore on his foot. It got infected. Very painful. The sore never healed.

He took to drinking & smoking weed. To help him relax. I think. Then he went into the hospital for pneumonia. They told him he was in renal failure.

His kidneys were functioning at 22%. He started dialysis. He began to care about his life then. He had waited too long. He did dialysis for three years.

4-hour sessions, every three days. He never complained. I would often find him in tears. He always pulled through, it seemed. He was doing so much better.

The world looked happier to him, he would say. It was the morning of April 15th. We found him dead in his bedroom. Two months short of his 26th birthday.

I miss him.

A Cyborg's Father

Syl, like most young children, is a storyteller. She likes to flip open our *Guide to North American Wildflowers* and concoct stories about her aunt's dog, Jenkins, while looking at illustrations of white trillium and squirrel corn. She introduces her stuffed animals to the characters that populate the books she loves; they set off on adventures together, sometimes inside of the book, but often beyond the confines of the binding. She will pluck a character off the page and cradle it, set it in her lap. A plush bear milks a paper cow. A young witch magics a swimming pool. I find myself asking her who and what she is: she might answer dog, or cat, or monkey, or Slobar, or even, in one instance, a pile of horse shit (poop, in her words). Physical and imaginary for her read as one continuous text; everything is fluid, merged, boundaryless.

In "A Cyborg Manifesto," Donna Haraway proposes a world (a future, a present) in which a non-binary fluidity is the norm. Boundaries between the human and its relation to machine, species, gender, the physical and non-physical realms, have fallen away. In her work, the evolutionary truth that the human form has never been distinct from the nonhuman world creates a more varied and unified definition of how it means to be a human, of how it means to be a cyborg.

This definition of the cyborg admittedly takes a moment to wrap the head around. Popular depictions of cyborgism have trained us toward the sci-fi grotesque: flesh and machine mashed together, awkward entanglements of wire and vein, metal and bone. Darth Vader, Robocop, Seven of Nine: these fictional borgs trigger both attraction and disgust; a fascination with how the body might be repurposed; repulsion at how inhuman their transformations have rendered them.

Fantastical future imaginings make for fun stories, but as a father (not of the Darth Vader variety, I hope) I find Haraway's practical cyborgism far more enticing. Here the cyborg is not a centuries-distant mash-up of parts but a reckoning with what bodies and tools and stories are at hand in the current moment: the nonhuman/human tools that are available to expand life, to allow that life a fuller realization, to simply keep that life alive.

I have begun to understand myself as a question, as a fluid part of Syl's extended cyborgism, as one microchip in the machinery that maintains her health and existence. I am the timekeeper. Measuring out days between device changes. Measuring out hours between insulin boluses, counting down the minutes until she needs to begin eating. Counting out the minutes until the juice kicks in to correct her lows. I have never loved time; now I find myself acutely attuned to it. I have never loved numbers; now I find myself always counting.

Questions lead to stories. Let us make a story together. Let us sit on the floor and weave a tale of bears, insects, numbers, machines, people.

◊

What Haraway's vision/metaphor of the cyborg pushes us toward is not a world that might scan like a Philip K. Dick novel, populated with undercover androids and autonomous eyeballs, but rather a way of reseeing what is already present. Haraway terms this speculative fabulation, a type of narration that enables new takes on what is already possible. Not in the sense of pure invention, but in enlarging the spectrum of perception. What stories have always been present that simply haven't been told? How might we unfold the complicated origami of history to reveal the unspoken relationships that will remake the future? How do we begin to denormalize human existence through observational reimagining like Eva Hayward's "fingeryeyes," which offers up a study of cup corals as "an act of sensuous manifesting," a "reading of how making sense and sensual meaning are produced through determinable and permeable species boundaries."[1]

In my mind I watch a scrambled timeline flicker past, a sketched narrative of my life: it appears nebulous, but not porous. Have I made room for the potentiality of cup corals? What spaces and species have I failed to consider, to let in? What other lives have I not seen, not entered into? I am reminded of the documentary *My Octopus Teacher,* in which filmmaker Craig Foster forges a bond with an octopus living in a kelp forest off the coast of South Africa, an interspecies relationship that wrenches him out of the dark narcissism of human existence. In an other form of life he finds a pathway out of personal void, a return to a creative narrative. He realizes, submerged in the ocean's violent music, an imaginal portal into the realm of the living.

◊

Medical cyborgism is an effort of fabulation. The bad days, the worst cases, the failed technologies, the ever-evolving, ever-

---

1 Eva Hayward, "FINGERYEYES: Impressions of Cup Corals," *Cultural Anthropology* 25, no. 4 (2010): 577.

perplexing relationship between machine and body: we build stories to make sense of what makes no sense, to keep ourselves going, to mash up the real and pure speculation. Narratives constructed from unanswerable questions: Why, for no discernable reason, did Syl's blood sugar soar into the 300s? Why are her ketones so elevated when she seems perfectly healthy? Why did her CGM fail? Before Syl's diagnosis, I had always considered medicine a scientific endeavor, a process of elimination. Now I see it is a storyteller's craft, ever circling the unknown, a melodrama of resolution and crisis.

For all that chronic illness strips away (spontaneity, relaxation, sleep), it gives back in the way it craters perception. Solid ground is but another myth. When I watch Syl tell the story of her illness, when I see her pretend to change her fuzzy turtle's insulin pump or draw blood from a teddy bear paw, every time I am newly heartbroken, a lump of sandstone washed through again and again, left on the brink of crumbling.

Holes waiting to be occupied. Passed through. Felt.

◊

Haraway writes that for cyborgs, "fathers, after all, are inessential."[2] When I first encountered this sentence my sense of self stuttered, strobed, flashed out of sight.

And yet this is Haraway's point exactly: it is the cyborg's natural inclination to change the point of view from which the story is told. In human history fathers have been the storytellers, have shaped the world with their narratives. Reductive, racist, misogynistic, narcissistic, power-hungry fabulations. Cyborgs, who often find no version of themselves in these Anglo-Darwinist and patriarchal tales, who, because they understand inter-

---

2 Donna J. Haraway, "A Cyborg Manifesto," In *Manifestly Haraway* (Minneapolis: University of Minnesota Press, 2016), 10.

dependence as necessary for life, must as a means of survival shrug these stories off. They are the storytellers who will shape the human future, which can only be an extra-human future.

Like a song, this thought holds me together.

Bibliography

"All Is Full of Love." *Björk Wiki.* https://björk.fandom.com/wiki/All_Is_Full_of_Love_(song).
Alighieri, Dante. *Inferno.* Translated by Mary Jo Bang. Minneapolis: Graywolf Press, 2012.
Barnett, Richard. "Diabetes." *The Lancet* 375, no. 9710 (2010): 191. DOI: 10.1016/S0140-6736(10)60079-7.
Bechdel, Alison. *The Secret to Superhuman Strength.* New York: Houghton Mifflin Harcourt, 2021.
Benner, Scott. Episode 252. *Juicebox Podcast,* August 12, 2019. https://www.juiceboxpodcast.com/episodes/jbp252.
Berninger, Matt. *Broken Record Podcast,* May 2, 2023. https://www.pushkin.fm/podcasts/broken-record/matt-berninger.
Björk. *All Is Full of Love* (US CD single). Elektra Records, 1999.
Bloom, Madison. "Holly Herndon Announces New Album *PROTO*." *Pitchfork,* March 11, 2019. https://pitchfork.com/news/holly-herndon-announces-new-album-proto-shares-video-watch.
Boyer, Anne. *The Undying.* New York: Picador, 2019.
Brady, Andrea. "Alternative Arrangements." *FENCE.* https://fenceportal.org/alternative-arrangements/.
Brennan, David John. *Murder Ballads: Exhuming the Body Buried beneath Wordsworth's Lyrical Ballads.* Earth: punctum books, 2016.

Centers for Disease Control & Prevention. "National Diabetes Statistics Report." 2020. https://www.cdc.gov/diabetes/pdfs/data/statistics/national-diabetes-statistics-report.pdf.

Choi, Franny. *Soft Science.* Farmington: Alice James Books, 2019.

———. "What a Cyborg Wants." *Waxwing Magazine* 15 (2018). https://waxwingmag.org/items/issue15/21_Choi-What-a-Cyborg-Wants.php.

Chong, Celeste. "History of the BodyTalk System." *The Inside Job,* December 16, 2019. https://theinsidejob.sg/history-of-bodytalk-system.

Christian, M. "How SexyCyborg's Light Up Breast Implants Celebrate the Artificial." *Future of Sex,* March 11, 2020. https://futureofsex.net/augmentation/how-sexycyborgs-light-up-breast-implants-celebrate-the-artificial.

Fink, Joseph. "Kevin's Law Makes 72-hour Supply of More Medication Available to Patients." *Pharmacy Times* 87, no. 10 (2021): 54. https://www.pharmacytimes.com/view/kevin-s-law-makes-72-hour-supply-of-more-medication-available-to-patients.

Haraway, Donna J. "A Cyborg Manifesto." In *Manifestly Haraway,* 5–68. Minneapolis: University of Minnesota Press, 2016.

———. *Staying with the Trouble: Making Kin in the Chthulucene.* Durham: Duke University Press, 2016.

Hayward, Eva. "FINGERYEYES: Impressions of Cup Corals." *Cultural Anthropology* 25, no. 4 (2010): 577–99. DOI: 10.1111/j.1548-1360.2010.01070.x.

Herndon, Holly. "Holly Herndon – Birthing PROTO." *YouTube,* September 10, 2019. https://www.youtube.com/watch?v=v_4UqpUmMkg.

Herndon, Holly (as told to Andy Beta). "Inside the World's First Mainstream Album Made with AI." *Vulture,* November 13, 2019. https://www.vulture.com/2019/11/holly-herndon-on-proto-an-album-made-with-ai.html.

Hernon, Matthew. "Why Is Japan Still Biased against People with Disabilities?" *Tokyo Weekender,* July 11, 2017. https://

www.tokyoweekender.com/art_and_culture/japanese-culture/why-is-japan-still-biased-against-people-with-disabilities/.

"Hunter." *Björk & Family Tree*. http://bjorknet.altervista.org/restored/10/.

"Japanese Man Who Killed 19 Disabled People Sentenced to Death." *BBC News*, March 16, 2020. https://www.bbc.com/news/world-asia-51903289.

Jessica. "Progress Report: Robyn." *Stereogum*. March 10, 2010, https://www.stereogum.com/292372/progress-report-robyn/interviews/progress-report/.

Kierkegaard, Søren. *The Essential Kierkegaard*. Edited and translated by Howard Hong and Edna Hong. Princeton: Princeton University Press, 2000.

Koestenbaum, Wayne. "On Panic: Whose Woods These Are I Think I Know." *Poetry Foundation*, July 3, 2023. https://www.poetryfoundation.org/poetrymagazine/articles/160534/on-panic-whose-woods-these-are-i-think-i-know.

McRuer, Robert. *Crip Theory: Cultural Signs of Queerness and Disability*. New York: NYU Press, 2006.

Moran, Michael. "Sexy 'Human Cyborg' Plans Give Mankind an Upgrade as She Shows Off Fiber Optic Glowing Boobs." *Daily Star*, April 17, 2020. https://www.dailystar.co.uk/news/latest-news/sexy-human-cyborg-plans-give-21821712.

Shelborne, Philip. "Björk's Homogenic Album Review." *Pitchfork*, February 5, 2017. https://pitchfork.com/reviews/albums/22835-homogenic.

Shelley, Mary. *Frankenstein or The Modern Prometheus*. Cambridge: MIT Press, 2017. DOI: 10.7551/mitpress/10815.001.0001.

"The Always Uncjorked Björk!" Interview with John Savage. *Interview Magazine* (1995). http://bjork.fr/Interview-1995,982.

Tolentino, Jia. *Trick Mirror*. New York: Random House, 2019.

Turrell, James. *Roden Crater*. https://rodencrater.com/about.

Vitale, Anna. *Our Rimbaud Mask*. Brooklyn: Ugly Duckling Presse, 2018.

Wang, Xiaowei. *Blockchain Chicken Farm*. New York: Farrar, Straus and Giroux, 2020.

Watson, Rebecca. "Vice vs. Sexy Cyborg: How US Journalists Nearly Ruined a Chinese Maker." *Skepchick,* April 16, 2018. https://skepchick.org/2018/04/vice-vs-sexy-cyborg-us-journalists-nearly-ruined-chinese-maker.

Weise, Jillian. *Cyborg Detective*. Rochester: BOA Editions, 2019.

Wu, Naomi. "Shenzhen Tech Girl Naomi Wu, Part 3: Defunding, Deplatforming, and Detention." *Medium,* November 7, 2019. https://medium.com/@therealsexycyborg/shenzhen-tech-girl-naomi-wu-part-3-defunding-deplatforming-and-detention-140fed4b9554.

www.ingramcontent.com/pod-product-compliance
Lightning Source LLC
Chambersburg PA
CBHW072045160426
43197CB00014B/2630